THE
EVERYTHING®
BABY SHOWER BOOK

2nd Edition

Throw a memorable event for the mother-to-be

Sabrina Hill and Joni Russell

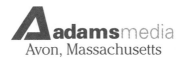

▲adamsmedia
Avon, Massachusetts

With Much Love to Our Families: David, Ashleigh, Kevin, and Chelcie Hill. And to Lloyd, Josh, Jen, Haley, and Lauren Russell, and Meredith and Nate Snyder. And to Dad, Irving Schoenfeld. Your love and support mean "everything" to us.

An Everything® Series Book.
Everything® and everything.com® are registered trademarks of F+W Publications, Inc.

Published by Adams Media, an F+W Publications Company
57 Littlefield Street, Avon, MA 02322 U.S.A.
www.adamsmedia.com

ISBN 10: 1-59869-552-5
ISBN 13: 978-1-59869-552-6

Printed in the United States of America.

J   I   H   G   F   E   D   C   B   A

Library of Congress Cataloging-in-Publication Data
is available from the publisher.

This publication is designed to provide accurate and authoritative information with regard to the subject matter covered. It is sold with the understanding that the publisher is not engaged in rendering legal, accounting, or other professional advice. If legal advice or other expert assistance is required, the services of a competent professional person should be sought.

—From a *Declaration of Principles* jointly adopted by a Committee of the American Bar Association and a Committee of Publishers and Associations

Interior illustrations by Michelle Dorenkamp.

Many of the designations used by manufacturers and sellers to distinguish their products are claimed as trademarks. Where those designations appear in this book and Adams Media was aware of a trademark claim, the designations have been printed with initial capital letters.

This book is available at quantity discounts for bulk purchases.
For information, please call 1-800-289-0963.

Contents

Introduction / xiii

In the Beginning / 1
The Hostess's Responsibilities **2** • Special-Circumstance Showers **4** • Creating the Perfect Day to Say "Welcome Baby" **5** • When You're Planning Solo **7**

Planning Tools / 9
Hostess with the "Mostest" **10** • Setting a Date and Time **11** • Setting the Budget **12** • Planning Tips from Professional Experience **14** • Food and Beverage Needs **17** • Selecting a Great Location **18**

Creating a Theme / 25
Why Choose a Theme? **26** • Brainstorming the Shower Theme **27** • Turning Simple Ideas into Great Themes **29** • Themes from Movies, Television, and Pop Culture **30** • Fashionable Themes **31** • Gifts That Inspire Themes **33** • Going Themeless **34**

Invitations / 35
Who to Invite **36** • How to Invite **36** • What to Include on the Invitation **37** • Handling the R.S.V.P.s **38** • Creative Ideas for Invitations **39** • Adding Materials and Layers **42** • Special Delivery Options for Invitations **44**

5

The Art and Science of Menu Selection / **45**

Menu Basics **46** • Seating, Serving, and Style **46** • Basic Food Rules **48** • Name That Meal **49** • Food Rules **52** • Hostess in Labor **54** • When to Call the Caterer and When to Eat Out **55**

6

Décor and Favors / **59**

Basic Elements of Décor **60** • Baby Shower Color and Pattern Palettes **64** • Décor Ideas and Projects **66** • Clever Favors **69**

7

Fun and Games / **73**

Activities Versus Games **74** • Popular Shower Games **74** • Choosing an Activity or Game **76** • Activity 1: Setting-Up Baby-Massage Lessons **77** • Activity 2: Feeding Baby **78** • Baby Shower Arts and Crafts Activities **79** • Activity 3: Painted Canvas "Baby Quilt" **79** • Activity 4: Teddy Bear Workshop **80** • Activities That Create Moments and Memories **80** • Activity 5: Scrapbook-Making Shower **81** • Activity 6: Parenting-Advice Book **82** • Activity 7: Cards for Birthdays One to Twenty-One **82**

8

Presents and Accounted For / **83**

Gift-Giving 101 **84** • Finding the Newest Trends **85** • Tried-and-True Traditional Baby Gifts **87** • Gift Giving with a Theme **89** • Personalized Gifts **90** • The Gift Registry **91**

9

Celebrity-Style Baby Showers / **93**

Headline-Making Details **94** • THEME IDEA 1: Under Construction **95** • THEME IDEA 2: The Princess Wears Prada **99** • THEME IDEA 3: Roll Out the Red Carpet: A Celebrity-Style Couples Shower **103**

10 Girlfriends Go Wild Shower / 107

Who Can Use This Theme **108** • Setting Up at Home **108** • Setting Up Away from Home **108** • Invitation Ideas **109** • THEME IDEA 1: Playing Footsie, Tootsie! A Pedicure Shower **109** • THEME IDEA 2: Cute as a Button Shower **114** • THEME IDEA 3: Everything Night-Night Shower **116**

11 Zen Tea Shower / 119

Who Can Use This Theme **120** • Setting Up at Home **120** • Setting Up Away from Home **120** • THEME IDEA 1: Tranquili-Tea Baby Shower **121** • THEME IDEA 2: Belly Bump Shower **128** • THEME IDEA 3: Tea for Two Shower **131**

12 A Grandparents' Shower / 133

Who Can Use This Theme **134** • Setting Up at Home **135** • Setting Up Away from Home **135** • Menu Ideas **136** • Invitation Ideas **136** • Music and Entertainment **137** • THEME IDEA 1: Baby Libris—Start a Children's Book Collection **138** • THEME IDEA 2: Save a Bundle Shower **141**

13 Broadway Baby Shower: For Drama Buffs and Drama Queens / 145

Who Can Use This Theme **146** • Setting Up at Home **146** • Setting Up Away from Home **147** • Menu Ideas and Options **147** • Invitation Ideas and Script **148** • THEME IDEA 1: *Mamma Mia:* A Shower and Musical Review for Couples **149** • THEME IDEA 2: *Hello, Dolly!* Welcoming the Newest Star **151** • THEME IDEA 3: Baby Grand: A Piano-Bar Sing-Along Shower **154**

14 Jack and Jill Showers for Couples / 157

Who Can Use This Theme **158** • THEME IDEA 1: Diapers Wild! A Poker Party and Shower **158** • THEME IDEA 2: Lucky Strike! From Bowling Pins to Diaper Pins **162** • THEME IDEA 3: The La Maze–Le Mans Car-Seat Rally **165**

15 Being Neighborly Showers / 169

Who Can Use This Theme **170** • THEME IDEA 1: Red Wagon Progressive Shower **170** • THEME IDEA 2: The Red Wagon Food Challenge Shower **174** • THEME IDEA 3: The Red Wagon Community Diaper Drive **179**

16 Showers for Dads / 183

Who Can Use This Theme **184** • Setting Up at Home **184** • Setting Up Away from Home **185** • Invitation Ideas **185** • THEME IDEA 1: Daddies in the Digital Age **186** • THEME IDEA 2: Extreme Nursery Makeover **190** • THEME IDEA 3: Tailgate Shower **193**

17 Showers for Urban Über-Babes / 197

Who Can Use This Theme **198** • Setting Up at Home **198** • Setting Up Away from Home **199** • Invitation Ideas and Script **199** • THEME IDEA 1: Phat and Phabulous: The Maternity Girl's a Fashionista **200** • THEME IDEA 2: Maternity Girl Goes Tourista **203** • THEME IDEA 3: The Maternity Girl's Guide to Urban Artistas **206**

18 e-Showers: From Virtual to Desktop to "Lap-Top" / 209

Who Can Use This Theme **210** • THEME IDEA 1: The Virtually Virtual Shower **210** • THEME IDEA 2: The Desktop Shower: Coffee-Break Contractions **213** • THEME IDEA 3: The "Lap-Top" Shower Visit **217** • Celebrating a New Bundle of Joy **220**

19 Shower Recipes / 221

Recipes and Ideas **222** • Chapter 9: Celebrity-Style Showers **222** • Chapter 10: Girlfriends Go Wild Showers **235** • Chapter 11: Zen Tea Showers **240** • Chapter 12: Grandparents' Showers **247** • Chapter 13: Broadway Baby Showers **250** • Chapter 14: Jack and Jill Showers for Couples **252** • Chapter 15: Being Neighborly Showers **256** • Chapter 16: Showers for Dads **261** • Chapter 18: e-Showers **268**

Appendix A: Resources / 275

Appendix B: Project Directions / 285

Appendix C: Templates for Customized Printing Projects / 289

Index / 291

Acknowledgments

LIKE THE BABIES these showers celebrate, a book requires care, nurturing, and expertise to be born. This book was no exception; it was the result of work and input from many loving hands.

To our first-round editor, Lloyd, who added and subtracted commas, hyphenated and colon-ed phrases, and corrected innumerable spelling errors—our second-round editors have no idea how much trouble you saved them.

To Ashleigh Hill, Chelcie Hill, and Hilary Norcott, who fact-checked and formatted every chapter.

To our agent, Andrea Hurst, who matched us to this project and expertly guided us through the publishing experience.

To our editor, Kerry Smith, for her patience and encouragement.

To our development editor, Brett Palana-Shanahan, who brought us from the words on a page to a book on the shelf.

To the entire staff of Los Gatos Coffee Roasting Company, especially Lorraine, Len, and Morgan, for two perfect cups of Sumatra/Ethiopian Blend and two sublime currant scones every morning (the only way to start a writing day in our opinion), and to John and Faun at the Los Gatos Gourmet for the picnic-style lunches we ate desk-side so we could continue to make deadlines.

To our children and their spouses, who accommodated our writing schedules, stuffed envelopes, and shared in the ups and downs of authorship.

To our husbands, David and Lloyd, who read, reread, and reread again the many drafts of our work. Your critiques, financial support, and confidence in us got us through this process.

Top Ten Baby Shower Myths
Busted in this Book

1. Baby showers are for women only.

Not so! Baby shower fun is dictated by the activities, not the gender of the guests.

Anything from tailgating to a scavenger hunt can become a shower idea.

2. Baby showers are only for moms-to-be.

False. You can throw a shower for a dad-to-be, a grandparent-to-be,

or a sibling-to-be.

3. Baby showers should be limited to one per pregnancy.

Not true. You can throw more than one shower for someone, but don't expect

repeat guests to bring a gift to each shower.

4. Baby shower guests don't expect thank yous from the guest of honor.

Thank yous are required and appreciated.

5. Baby shower guests don't want to see the presents opened.

Not true. Guests have put thought into buying their presents and should see

them opened.

6. Baby shower games are dumb.

Games and activities get guests involved. Pick games that suit the interests

of your guests.

7. Baby shower themes should be old-fashioned.

Times change! Make use of trendy ideas and pop culture to keep your shower

fresh and modern.

8. Baby shower gifts must be selected from the gift registry.

Not necessarily. The gift registry is a convenience, not a requirement.

9. Baby showers should be held in a home.

Not so! You can throw a shower almost any place!

10. Baby showers should be big events.

False. If mom-to-be can't come out to play, you can bring a small

shower right to her bedroom.

Introduction

▶ BABIES. THEY'RE IRRESISTIBLE. And their arrival is a cause for celebration whether they're the first or the fourteenth. When they're the first, you need a lot of equipment and advice, and when they're the fourteenth, you need a lot of help and support! One thing is certain, you need a party! This book celebrates the baby shower in all its forms and renditions. It also celebrates the shower hostess or hostesses. Your job is to create the kind of party that not only welcomes the baby but also welcomes the guests. Here you'll find ideas that you can copy as is or modify to add your own polish and panache.

The baby shower was born in the late 1800s. In its infancy, showers were given after the baby was born because it was not considered fashionable for pregnant women to be seen in public. So Victorian ladies gathered for tea after the baby was born to bestow upon the little cherub handmade or silver gifts.

Wow, have times changed! Today, baby shower planning starts as soon as the blue plus sign appears on the home pregnancy test. Guest lists include boyfriends, girlfriends, and husbands, children and pets, coworkers, family, and neighbors. Showers come in the form of cocktail parties, barbeques, and sporting events, as well as the traditional teas and garden parties. You'll attend them in homes and hotels, backyards and bowling alleys, restaurants and wine bars, and beaches and billiards rooms.

The modern hostess or host (yes, men can give a shower) doesn't face the restrictions imposed from years past. Almost any party ideas can be transformed into a baby shower. And they aren't just for moms and babies anymore, either. Husbands can throw a shower for their brother or best friend at a ballgame or over a hand of poker, and this book takes you through every step from menu selection to printing favor labels from your computer.

Shower invitations have also turned away from the traditional fuzzy pink bunnies, yellow duckies, and powder-blue rattles stuck unceremoniously onto cardstock. While custom or preprinted cards are still the most popular way to get the word out, electronic invitations are proving to be a force to be "invited with." With a silver tongue and a few keystrokes, guests can get the "411" about the party delivered right to their hand-held PDA.

The gifts have changed, too! Though a handmade blanket or sweater is always sought after, the gift list has expanded to include jogging strollers, cribs, bedding, baby juicers, and more. New equipment has spawned a new vocabulary—co-sleepers, Pack 'n Plays, Boppys, binkies, Robeez, Pee-pee Teepees, and kangaroo pouches. Baby gift giving is now a multimillion dollar industry! Department stores have opened gift registries to ensure that babies get what they need. Within these pages you will find a plethora of ideas for giving group gifts, creating personalized treasures, and bestowing the ultimate gifts of time, friendship, and extra sets of hands.

Whether you mix and match ideas to create your own unique affair or you grab a theme and follow it to the letter, the most important element to the entire planning process is to enjoy the good fortune of a friend or family member and have some fun. A baby shower should be a joyous celebration of all the optimism and good wishes we offer up to new parents and the new life they are bringing to share with us. So let the planning begin!

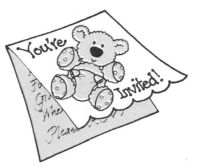

Chapter 1

In the Beginning

WHEN YOUR BEST FRIEND, sister, sister-in-law, neighbor, or coworker calls you with the exciting news that she is having a baby, you know you have an important job to do: planning the baby shower! Should you throw a shower? Should you plan it alone? Who should you invite? When should you have it? What should you serve? How should you decorate? Should dads or husbands be invited? Should alcohol be served? Should the shower wait until the baby has arrived? With a "should" in every question, what should a shower-thrower do?

The Hostess's Responsibilities

Traditionally, only friends threw the mommy-to-be a shower, not family. While it is now considered acceptable for a sister, sister-in-law, cousin, or aunt to act as a hostess, according to etiquette experts, it is usually not considered proper form for a mother or mother-in-law to host such an event.

E-FACT

If you choose to throw a surprise shower, you will need an accomplice—preferably a close friend, family member, or spouse who can keep a secret and has a good poker face! Let guests know on the invitation that the secret must be kept. Also be sure to make special parking arrangements—a dozen cars in the driveway is a dead giveaway that a party's afoot!

The shower guests of honor are the mommy-to-be and her baby. As guest of honor, her responsibilities are to arrive at the appointed hour, be as gracious and charming as possible and to accept with gratitude the gift of the shower and the array of presents and good wishes she will receive. As the hostess, you have responsibilities, too. You should consult with the mommy-to-be (unless it's a surprise) to give her a range of dates, tell her the maximum number of guests your home or budget will accommodate, and find out if there are any dietary considerations you should know about. You should also find out where she is registered for baby gifts (if she is). Beyond that, it is your job to plan and arrange the party and her job to be a good guest of honor.

Though most American baby showers are held prior to the baby's birth, there is nothing wrong with having one early in the pregnancy or after the baby arrives. There are advantages to both. If you are planning one ahead of the due date, the new parents will have a chance to relax and enjoy the party and be able to unwrap and put away the wonderful presents without the interruption of feedings, diapers, and sleeplessness. Showers held after the baby's birth have the very distinct upside of knowing the baby's gender, size, and name.

Shower Essentials

Most showers take place over two to four hours and include refreshments—ranging from tea and biscuits to a meal with dessert—games or an activity, and gift giving and opening. Use this as a general guideline as you begin gathering the information you will need to party plan.

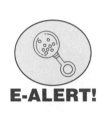

E-ALERT!

Unfortunately, there is a new trend to forego opening gifts at a party. However, since guests have taken the time to shop, select, purchase, wrap, and carry a gift to the party, it is only natural that they would want to see the reaction upon opening the present. Allow time for the guest of honor to open each gift and acknowledge the giver "in the moment."

The guest list may be determined by default—all the people in a certain group, such as work colleagues, will be invited. It may be determined by geography—all the neighbors in the cul-de-sac—or by social group. Whatever the case, the size and makeup of the guest list will determine many of the party's details. One thing to consider when embarking on this planning endeavor is to make sure that no one in any guest group is excluded on purpose. It is easy enough to squeeze in one or two extras rather than deal with a lifetime of hurt feelings.

Important Shower Know-How

Because today's new mothers-in-waiting may be in the workforce, belong to a religious or social group, be involved with the activities of school-aged children, and so on, it is possible that more than one group may wish to plan a shower. That's great, as long as guests are not expected (or required) to bring a present to each party.

Several baby shower Web sites and articles have indicated that it is alright to excuse the new mom-to-be from writing thank-you notes for shower gifts. They are wrong. Ask any etiquette expert, from Amy

Vanderbilt to Emily Post—thank-you notes are a must. No one expects a two-page report from a new mother, but a brief, gracious acknowledgment is required.

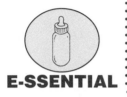

E-SSENTIAL

As hostess, make the new mommy's life a little easier by addressing thank-you notes at the shower! Have a package of notes on hand at the shower. Give an envelope to each guest and ask her to write her name and address on the front. Gather them in a bag, ready for writing and mailing.

Special-Circumstance Showers

Babies come to a family in a variety of ways and often at unpredictable times. Your philosophy should be simply to welcome every baby by celebrating the arrival at whatever time will work for the new parents. The same rules for planning the perfect shower apply, regardless of when and how the baby gets there. It is a wise shower-thrower who has a "Wrap everything up for later; she's in labor!" attitude. There are no special rules if the shower is for an adopted child or surrogate birth, except to come and celebrate a new life!

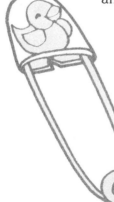

It's a very special circumstance indeed if a new mother is expecting more than one baby, but it doesn't change the shower planning one bit. You simply plan for more babies! It is also a good idea to choose an earlier shower date, as multiple babies often arrive early. Location can be another consideration when more than one bundle is on the way. Moms may not be able to travel or sit for long periods, or may even be confined to a bed or hospital. Be flexible, keep it simple, and make it portable—your shower will be just perfect wherever and whenever it takes place.

Creating the Perfect Day to Say "Welcome Baby"

Parties, like people, need good bones. They provide a solid structure for everything else to be built on. Every party has similar bone structure, with slight variations to accommodate the type of occasion you are celebrating. Baby showers are no exception.

Every party has a beginning, a middle filled with party layers, and an end. If you plan around this framework, your party is sure to be a hit.

The Beginning: Invitation and Welcome

For your guests, the party begins when the invitation arrives. It sets the tone, hints at the style, may introduce the theme, and gives the guests the party's vital statistics. Most importantly, it gets people excited about coming to the shower!

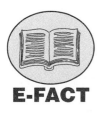

E-FACT

Set up a manned "Welcome Station" near the entrance of your home (or party room, if away from home). Have a cocktail or beverage, a nametag, and an itinerary (if there is one) ready for guests as they arrive. It says "welcome" in a big way, and sets a party tone for the rest of the shower.

Once the appointed day and time arrive, the invitation is a thing of the past. Now it's up to you, the hostess, to set the party in motion. How do you do it? Be prepared to greet the guests—actually open the door, shake their hands, lock them in a warm embrace, and even compliment their shoes. Welcome them into your home and say, "I'm so glad you're here!" While it is often chaotic at the moment the guests arrive, make a concerted effort to practice this welcoming ritual. You will be surprised at the positive effect this single gesture has on your occasion.

When all (or most) of the guests have arrived, the hostess(es) must officially begin the festivities. While it's nice to try to give everyone a beverage before the introductions, don't delay or forego this important moment. You are the party cruise director. Assemble the group, and let them know who's who and what's coming. If the group is unacquainted, ask each guest to introduce herself and tell how she knows the mommy-to-be. Taking the time to introduce or reacquaint the guests is not only a great icebreaker, but a perfect note to start your party on.

The Middle: The Party Layers

Once you have gone through introductions and welcomes, people will be on the move—after all, it's a party. Every shower will have its own specific layers that will make it unique and fun, regardless of your style, budget, or venue.

- ✓ **Tummy fillers.** You can serve cake and ice cream or a lavish five-course dinner, but you should serve something.
- ✓ **Décor.** It can be as simple as decorative napkins and party plates or as elaborate as flowers, candles, and a pink or blue silk-swathed tent. Make the day special with a touch of décor.
- ✓ **Music.** Music adds an energizing layer to the party. Unless you are having the shower in your cubicle or a library, bring an iPod, portable stereo, a guitarist, an orchestra—whatever suits your style and budget.
- ✓ **Conversation opportunities.** Your introductions have opened the door to great conversation. Now give your guests some time to talk before rushing them on to games, activities, or entertainment.
- ✓ **Game, activity, or entertainment.** This gives guests a chance to interact and to share an experience. Showers have a built-in activity—the present opening; however, there is no rule against having another one. Pick something you know your particular group will enjoy.

The End: Goodbyes, Good Wishes, and Thank Yous

At a baby shower, when the last gift is opened, it is usually the signal that the party's over. The mommy-to-be should take a moment to thank the guests for coming and the hostess(es) for throwing such a lovely shower.

She and the hostess should help guests with coats, favors, and goodbyes. If a guest leaves early, the hostess should walk them to the door and thank them for coming. This simple gesture is as important as the welcoming greeting.

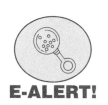

E-ALERT!

The shower's guest of honor will want to thank guests for attending her party and will also write notes of thanks for gifts, but the hostess must also thank guests for attending. A simple announcement of gratitude as the party winds down is a gracious finishing touch.

When You're Planning Solo

The decision to plan a shower alone or with a group will depend on myriad factors—geography, budget, time, desire, expectations—and you know best what will work for you. The tradition of bestowing showers varies around the country in social communities, family situations, and business environments. If you have decided to plan the shower alone, let your effort be the labor of love intended by following this advice:

✓ **Keep size and budget within your means.** If you're hoping to do all the work yourself, keep it small and simple. If your budget is expansive—knock yourself out and hire help.

✓ **Enjoy the planning.** This is a party for a friend, not a survival game, so don't let yourself feel overwhelmed by the decisions. No one but you will know that you wanted hot-pink napkins but couldn't find them.

✓ **Allow extra time.** When possible, give yourself the gift of time. Use six weeks lead time instead of four. Making one party favor might seem simple, but making twenty by yourself will take longer than you may expect. Don't leave a lot of details for the week of the event.

✓ **Have a party slush fund.** Give yourself a small cash fund for use in the days before the party. If you do run out of time to make the centerpieces, you'll have some cash to run to the local florist.

When You're Planning a Shower by Committee

There is nothing wrong with planning a shower alone, but there are some distinct advantages to planning a shower with a group. Sharing the work and responsibilities with family, friends, or coworkers can lighten the load and increase the fun factor. You will be able to draw on the skills and expertise of the group; maybe one of you is a fabulous cook, or an invitation artist, or a floral designer. Plan to make use of the particular strengths and interests of each shower-thrower. Everyone who wants to should be able to participate in the planning, staging, and preparation of the party.

Communication is the critical, pivotal piece when it comes to planning a shower by committee. If your fellow shower-throwers are in the same area, get together to discuss and plan the details. If not, have a phone meeting, conference call, even an online chat with the group. As a group, determine the shower theme (see Chapter 3) and *who* will handle *what*, from food to décor to invitations, and the like. You should also appoint someone as the point-of-contact person. She will be responsible for making sure that as you move forward, everyone has received the most up-to-date information regarding the shower and that nobody gets left out. Plan to stay in touch throughout the planning process and schedule a meeting or phone call during the week of the event to catch up on any last-minute details and changes.

The point person should keep a working list of the shower details and responsibilities and each cohost should have a copy. Including cohosts in all aspects of the planning is so important to the outcome of the party. It may take a little more time and a little more effort, but the results will be well worth this extra attention. Brainstorming a theme and how to accomplish it is a great excuse to get together, have some laughs, and pull the party details into focus as a group.

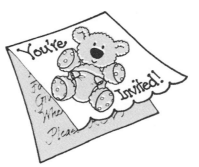

Chapter 2

Planning Tools

PLANNING A BABY SHOWER is no different from planning any other type of party. There is some basic information that must be gathered to determine how you will proceed. Whether this is your first baby shower or you're a shower-throwing veteran, one thing remains constant: The entire reason for this activity is to shower the new baby and new mommy with love and good wishes—and an occasional present is also nice. Ultimately, your task as planner is to create a relaxed and welcoming environment where these sentiments can be expressed.

Hostess with the "Mostest"

Hosting a baby shower doesn't have to be a lot of work, and it doesn't have to cost a lot of money. It should, however, be fun to plan. As with any job, the same results can be achieved with many different tools. You may find that a binder or BlackBerry suits your needs, or perhaps Post-its on your refrigerator work best. Those idiosyncrasies will define your record-keeping style and may also define the style of the shower. Use what works for you to your advantage. Don't fight it, celebrate it!

Party-Planning Basics

Entertaining is the marriage of your party vision with the needs of your guests. Before you begin organizing and selecting the details, stop for a moment and create a mental picture of the shower in your head. Is it a confection of gossamer-clad women with parasols at high tea on the veranda, high-heeled fashionistas sipping nonalcoholic Appletinis at a trendy restaurant, or dear old Grandma and all the cousins reminiscing on Aunt Betty's patio? There is no wrong answer—all of theses showers can be successful and fun. But you need to have an idea to shoot for, so think, think, think.

Three "Ds" of Decision Making

There are three things you should keep in mind when planning any party:

✓ **Demographics of guest group.** The demographics of the guest group or groups (coworkers, relatives, age group, gender mix) will help you narrow down the venue location and size, as well as the time of day and possibly the degree of formality.

✓ **Degree of formality.** For baby showers, this ranges from jeans at a barbeque to high tea at the Ritz. It is highly unusual to have a formal, black-tie baby shower. This factor may also be influenced by the location. A shower at work might be business casual, whereas a shower in your backyard might be jeans casual.

✓ **Day of week/Time of day/Time of year.** Most baby showers are held in the last trimester, generally about six to eight weeks before the baby's due date. This factor obviously will determine any seasonal influence on your event, such as having it indoors or outside, using specific colors, and so on. If you are inviting work friends and social friends, you may choose an after-work or weekend time. If it's other young mothers, morning coffee with toddlers may be more appropriate. These time factors will influence several decisions, such as guest list and menu.

These three "Ds" can be assessed in a matter of minutes, but they are the cornerstones for the balance of the detail decisions. They should be part of the initial discussion when you are cohosting a shower with another person or with a group.

Setting a Date and Time

Which comes first, the venue or the date? Well, that depends. If you are having an at-home shower, date considerations depend on your own calendar and the guest of honor's due date. If you have chosen to have it at a restaurant, hotel, or other venue, be aware that you may need more lead time and some date flexibility. Hotels that are popular for weddings may not have much weekend availability—you may need months to book the date you want. Holiday and vacation seasons also present some scheduling challenges as your guests' calendars fill up with travel plans or social commitments.

Ideally, the mother-to-be or her spouse will be able to give you several dates that would work in her last trimester. As you narrow the date range down to a specific day, remember to take into account work schedules, commute or travel considerations, and naps or babysitting needs. If you do it during the day on a weekday, women who work will likely not be able to attend. Though you can't accommodate everyone's schedule, the goal is to make it convenient for the widest possible number of people to attend this special occasion.

Weekend showers are popular because they allow the maximum number of guests to attend with minimum impact to their hectic work-week schedules and stress. They also allow an opportunity for out-of-town guests to have travel time. If a weekend won't work, perhaps you need to reconsider the format of the shower. Maybe a mid-week dessert and coffee format will be a better fit and still allow you to host the event.

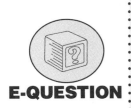

E-QUESTION

How long should a baby shower be?

At work: thirty minutes to one hour. Most at-work showers are held during a break or at lunch. At home: two to four hours. Coffee and dessert take less time than a meal or cocktail party. At a restaurant: two to three hours. Most restaurants set a start and end time and charge extra if your party runs late. Add an activity: one to two hours extra, depending on the activity.

Setting the Budget

Even if you've decided that the sky's the limit for the shower you're about to plan, you will then need to define "the sky." Every shower has a bottom line. The question is: How much money can you spend on this event? Protect yourself and your cohostess from shower sticker shock by putting it down on paper first, while there's still time to say, "No thanks, let's skip the caviar." Be realistic, and then get moving—you have a party to plan!

Budget Basics

While your plans for the baby shower will be unique and personalized, the main budget categories will be surprisingly similar. Most baby showers will include food, drinks, décor, music, entertainment or games, and invitations. The cost of these items, when added together, will be your total budget. The largest expense category is food and beverage, which generally accounts for 40 to 50 percent of your budget; decorations require 25 percent; with most of the balance going toward games, music, or other entertainment. And don't forget 10 percent for incidentals. You should always have a miscellaneous category to cover all those little things that mean so much but cost so much more than you thought.

There are several ways to approach the issue of budget. If you have never planned a shower before, use the following worksheet to determine a preliminary budget. Is the total what you wanted or can afford to spend? If it is, move forward; if not, write your bottom-line budget number down and work backward.

Budget-Planning Worksheets

Shower Budget

Estimated Number of Guests:

Cost Breakdown

ITEM	ESTIMATED COST	ACTUAL COST
Site		
Invitations		
Postage		
Decorations		
Food		
Beverages		
Music/Entertainment		
Party Favors		
Party Games/Prizes		
Present for Mother-to-Be		
Photography/Video		
Cleanup		
Rentals		
Miscellaneous		
Total		
Cost per person		

Planning Tips from Professional Experience

When you strip away all the glitz and glamour of being a professional party planner, what you're left with is years of experience and lots of tips. There are no great secrets here, just some commonsense, practical advice, and lots of practice. Anything you can do to lighten the work load during the planning phase and ease the stress event week, will make you a more relaxed hostess, which is the goal.

Stress Savers

✓ **Enlist help.** There's no medal of honor for going it alone. If you have a cohost or many cohosts, delegate the tasks and share the responsibilities. Husbands, children, and neighbors can be vital resources when it comes to napkin folding, furniture rearranging, and ribbon tying. And their involvement makes them feel like a part of the party.

✓ **Enlist professional help.** Sure, you can clean the house, mow the lawn, or roll pigs-in-a-blanket by yourself, but if you have to give up a workday (or more) to do so, you might consider professional help. Hire a house cleaner for the morning, have a gardener do the lawn and flower beds, get help to serve and clean up, consider a caterer, or hire a florist.

✓ **Don't procrastinate.** The closer you get to the big day, the more things will pile up on your planning plate. Anything that can be done ahead will make you feel more in charge as the party approaches.

✓ **Don't overschedule yourself.** During the week of the event, make your schedule easier, not harder. Reschedule your dental hygiene appointment. Throw in a frozen lasagna, hand off your turn to drive carpool.

Money Savers

As the details of your shower begin to fall into place, you may discover the conscientious hostess's worst nightmare—expenses add up quickly! As tempting as it is to forego the budget, stay on track and keep it simple. Here are a few money-saving tips in some of the "big ticket" party areas.

Food Tips

Some ideas for saving money on your food budget include:

✓ **Appetizers.** These tiny morsels tend to be more labor intensive than a plated meal. If you're serving at home, keep the appetizers simple—a tray of olives, hummus dip with pita chips, or a silver bowl of spiced nuts; these will give guests something to pop in their mouths without breaking your budget. If your shower is catered or at a restaurant or hotel, you can serve one or two passed hors d'oeuvres or a fruit or cheese platter before the meal instead of a canapé smorgasbord. This will satisfy the need to nibble without spoiling appetites for the meal to come.

✓ **Main course.** Whether you're cooking or someone else is doing the honors, too many choices can be a food-budget nightmare. For an at-home lunch, make the menu simple—a main-course salad, some crusty bread, and the dessert. If you're away from home, the buffet is always a popular choice because it feels more casual, but beware—it may cost more. At a buffet, food portions are less controlled, so more food is necessary to accommodate the same number of people. When serving a plated meal, don't let the guest choose from the main menu—it can be a runaway train! Instead, give your guests menu options by preselecting two or three choices that fit into your budget. The venue will often print a special menu with just those options, which is an elegant touch.

✓ **Desserts.** A cake is part of the traditional shower fare, but it's not the only dessert option. If a fancy cake will break your budget, consider a tower of cupcakes, mini-brownie sundaes, or ice-cream sandwiches made with cookies.

Decorating and Entertainment Tips

Some money-saving tips for decorations and entertainment include:

✓ **Décor at home.** While it is sometimes tempting to use the impending event date as the target for a major remodel or redecorating—resist the urge. This will definitely add stress and money woes to your shower. Moreover, it's not necessary. The great news is that eclectic is in! Walk around your home, and see what you have with "party eyes." A mirror can become a tray, mismatched wineglasses can hold votives. The old silver teapot is the perfect vase for flowers. If you are willing to move your furniture a little, you can cozy-up a family room or living room by reconfiguring a few chairs. Borrow interesting serving pieces, extra silverware, or a beautiful water pitcher from your mother, sister, or friend—it's amazing what a few pieces used in a different way can do for your décor. The grocery store is another great source of décor—a wooden bowl full of lemons, a pedestal cake plate of pears, bunches of fresh herbs— all offer an affordable, and edible, alternative to flowers, plants, or paper decorations.

✓ **Décor away from home.** The best advice here is to select a venue that is good-looking to begin with. And though these types of venues may at first glance appear to cost more, you may find that you spend far less on decorations. Many sites will provide a bud vase centerpiece or votive candles, which may be entirely adequate. Don't rule out a fancier site until you have done the math.

✓ **Entertainment.** Whether home or away, showers have a built-in entertainment factor. Ooohing and aaahing over booties and blankets can take some time, so you don't have to get carried away with entertainers and circus acts. Music adds a much-needed layer to any party, so do plan to have something playing in the background, but don't drown out the opportunity for great conversation.

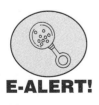

E-ALERT!

The gratuity and tax at restaurants, hotels, or through a caterer can add an additional 25–30 percent to the total bill for food and beverages. For a $40-per-person estimate, that's a whopping $12 more per person. It can be a budget buster if you haven't included it in your estimates. And by the way, a gratuity is not a tip; it is added automatically to your bill, whereas a tip is optional.

Time Savers

The more time you have, the more options you may have available to you. When you are out of time, you can incur rush charges for printing and mailing or extra labor charges to complete work in a shorter time frame. Some time-saving ideas include:

✓ **Plan ahead.** As you sail through the event week, think through the details and have a mental reheaseral of how the shower will look and what needs to be done to make your vision a reality.

✓ **Prepare ahead.** Somehow, the laws of time and space seem to collapse during the week of the event. Even with the best time management and planning, the favors that should take an hour to complete suddenly take two or more. Complete as many tasks as possible two weeks before the shower and keep those final days clear for "pop-up" problems.

✓ **Take one away.** It is a well-known rule of fashion that when you're finished getting dressed, look in the mirror and take one accessory away. It's the same for parties. During the final planning approach, take a critical look at what lies ahead and do a little editing. You won't miss the detail, but you will appreciate the extra time it will give you.

Food and Beverage Needs

At this stage in the party-planning game, it is very easy to get sidetracked with the yummy details of menu selection. Don't do it yet! All you need to know right this minute is what broad category of food you will be serving—breakfast, brunch, lunch, supper, dinner, coffee, cocktails—take your pick. Of course, it should correspond to the time of day, although "breakfast for dinner" or "desserts for breakfast" are fun ways to liven up the festivities.

There are always exceptions to the budget rule; however, following is a chart of some of the price ranges (based on dollars per person) for these mealtimes as a starting point for your budget worksheet.

Breakfast	$10 to $25
Brunch	$15 to $35
Coffee Break (at work)	$10 to $20
Lunch	$25 to $50
Dinner	$40 to $85 (can go higher depending on location)
Dessert and Coffee	$12 to $25
Cocktail-Party Food	$35 to $75

This information is based on national industry standards. If you live in a metropolitan area, prices may be higher. These prices do not include tax or gratuity. Gratuities range from 15 to 25 percent.

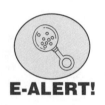

E-ALERT!

When considering a hotel or restaurant, remember that the posted catering menu does not include beverages unless specifically noted. Though some venues will include coffee and tea service, they may not include soft drinks, and they will not include alcoholic beverages.

Selecting a Great Location

The old real-estate adage is true in event planning: Location is everything. Choosing the venue is usually the first step in this phase. The right venue will set the tone for the event, making the management easier for the planner and allowing for greater control. For a shower, you will need a space to visit, a space to open presents, and a space to serve and eat. It's nice if you can get up and move from one area to another during the event; it allows for mingling and leg-stretching.

The Home Shower

A home is the classic backdrop for a baby shower. It's intimate, comfortable, and there's no pressure to get in and out on a time schedule. Having it at your house gives you plenty of flexibility, and it can sometimes save you money. If you have space for the number of guests expected, a reasonably convenient setup for food preparation, and access to adequate serving pieces (trays, coffee pots, etc.), a home shower may be the perfect choice for you.

If you decide a home shower is for you, there are many ways to adapt an *almost* perfect space into the *perfect* space, without an extreme makeover.

- ✓ **Rearrange furniture.** Reconfigure your space to allow for maximum seating and to open up floor space for better traffic flow.
- ✓ **Food stations.** Set up food and beverage stations around the house or yard. Create vignettes of seating and eating: Guests will enjoy a chance to engage in conversation in small groups.
- ✓ **Think inside-out.** If the weather allows, use a patio or backyard to fashion an outdoor room. Move indoor seating outside and group to form conversation areas.
- ✓ **Camouflage.** Who doesn't have a crayon-marked table or water-stained cushion? Colorful throws, tablecloths, a stack of books, magazines, or framed pictures can hide a multitude of blemishes.
- ✓ **Hide and seek.** When in doubt, gather unnecessary extras in a laundry basket and tuck out of sight. The party police won't catch you, promise.

The downside of hosting the shower at your house is that your house is in use, right up to the moment when you wave children and Dad off to the movies and dash upstairs to get dressed.

The responsibility of preparing the space for guests, as well as cleaning it all up afterward, is yours in addition to the rest of the shower-related preparations. Before you dive too deep into the hostessing pool, make sure that you have realistically evaluated what you need to stage the shower at your home. If you need to rent a tent, tables, chairs, umbrellas, dishes, and coffeepots and have to hire staff to assist you, compare the costs to that of a hotel or restaurant where those items are included.

The Hotel or Restaurant Shower

Choosing a hotel or restaurant for your shower can be a lot of fun. It's a good idea to look at several venues until you find the right one for you.

Many facilities now post pictures on their Web site, which can help you narrow the search before you even leave home. Be sure to look for a location that is convenient, has ample parking, adequate restroom facilities, and comfortable seating, and, of course, great food.

Once you've decided on a place, ask the manager to set aside the date in writing, preferably in the form of a contract. The contract should state the following things:

1. The date of the event
2. The start and end time of the party and the time allotted for setup and cleanup
3. The name of the room you have reserved for the party
4. The estimated cost of the party (or minimum cost of party)
5. The amount of deposit (usually 50 percent)
6. The due date for final payment and final guest count
7. The items and services included with the rental facility (i.e., linens, tables, chairs, candles, etc.)
8. The guarantee number
9. The cancellation policy
10. The "bumping" policy

Be a good businesswoman about this rental contract. Items 1–7 are fairly self-explanatory. Item 8, the guarantee, is the number of guests or minimum dollar amount that you are responsible for—regardless of how many people actually attend your party. Although you may like to estimate on the high side, in contract negotiation, you want to set a realistic number on the low side.

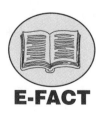

E-FACT

Hotels and restaurants can always accommodate small changes in the number of guests they can seat and serve, and in fact, most venues prepare for a 5–10 percent difference. When giving a guaranteed number of guests, take into account that there will always be last minute cancellations.

Item 9 relates to the cancellation policy. You want to be sure that if *any-thing* happens—the baby is early, you decide to do the shower elsewhere, etc.—you can get some or all of your deposit money back. Most places return some or all of your deposit if it is more than thirty days before the event.

Item 10 concerns the practice at some venues called "bumping." If a venue property has multiple party spaces, they may reserve the option to "bump" or move you to another room so that they may accommodate a larger party (or a group spending significantly more money) in the space you originally reserved. Though this situation is not usually the case for a baby shower, you should be aware of the venue's policy on this matter.

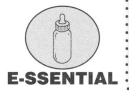

E-SSENTIAL

You have more negotiating options at a party venue than you may think if you are willing to be flexible. Breakfast, brunch, or lunch menus may offer a significant savings from a dinner menu. Work with the chef to create fewer courses, simpler service, or smaller portions to make your budget work.

Destination Showers

Many hostesses want to add an extra bit of panache to their shower event, so they opt for a destination shower. Locations that fall into this category are places like the beach or a specialty shop (a tea emporium, a wine shop, a clothing or baby boutique, etc.). These sites come with a bonus: The activity is built right in. There is also a trend toward hosting showers at day spas or nail salons. Treatments ranging from simple massages to manicures and pedicures are offered to guests.

If you have decided that you want to stage your shower in an unusual place, there are some special issues that you must consider. The first consideration is based on basic needs—is there shelter, are there restrooms, is it safe? A beach may be beautiful, but if the mother-to-be has to scale a cliff to get there, perhaps this isn't the best choice. Other considerations include food safety—is there a place to prepare, refrigerate, store, and dispose of food items? There may be restrictions about bringing food into a nail salon.

Does the site provide party essentials such as a room for guests to congregate in? Are tables and chairs available, or do they have to be rented?

Interesting places come with interesting challenges. They can work, but it's your responsibility to know exactly what those challenges will be before you sign anything. Also, do the math: That fabulous Japanese tea garden may be prettier than your own backyard, but if you need to rent furniture and linens to make it work, it may also be more expensive.

E-QUESTION

Can you use the venue's kitchen?
Some venues will give you access to their kitchen and some will connect you with their caterer. Most will not allow you to bring in your own food or cooking supplies, so make sure you know precisely what you'll be allowed to do before putting down a deposit.

If you have opted for a shower away from home, handle the booking like a professional. A site visit is a necessity. See for yourself what you're getting into. Don't count on someone else's recommendation alone. In order to get the most from your site visit:

✓ **Make an appointment.** You want to speak with the person who knows the property and handles both food and beverages.
✓ **Come prepared with questions.** This is the moment to ask all your questions. There are no dumb questions, so dig deep until you feel satisfied that you have enough information to make your decision.
✓ **Go with a friend.** You may be receiving a lot of information, and two heads are always better than one. Avoid taking small children or surly teenagers to the meeting; it can be distracting.

Venue Checklist

No matter which out-of-home venue you are thinking of, use the following checklist to help in your planning.

Does this venue work for the shower you want to plan?

○ What dates are available?
○ What space is available on those dates?
○ Is there indoor and outdoor space?
○ Can the room accommodate the service style you want? (i.e., buffet, food stations, sit-down)
○ Are there adequate restrooms for the number of guests?
○ Is there enough parking? Is there valet service? Is there any parking charge?
○ How will food and beverages be provided?
○ Who provides food and beverage service? Is it on-site? Catered?
○ What are the food and beverage minimums?
○ Will the event be adequately staffed? (ratio of servers to guests)

How does the site look?

○ What is the condition of the carpets and floors? Walls and drapes? Furniture and lighting?
○ What other amenities are available?
○ Do they have audio/visual equipment and staff available on-site?
○ Is there adequate power and lighting? Are there plugs available?

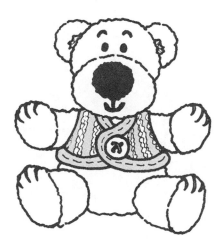

And finally . . .

○ Is there a Plan B for inclement weather, extra guests, food issues, etc?
○ Can the space be used in a different way in case of weather, change in party size, etc.?
○ Can you get a commitment in writing?

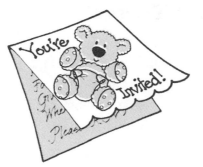

Chapter 3

Creating a Theme

A THEME MAKES A GATHERING FEEL LIKE A PARTY. Choosing a theme is an important element in the shower-planning process. It helps set the mood and tone for the party. It embodies the style and demonstrates the creativity of the hostess or cohostesses. And it adds a punch of fun to the festivities. This chapter will help spark some ideas for a creative, crowd-pleasing theme.

Why Choose a Theme?

When you select a shower theme, all the remaining choices will be influenced by this decision. Having a theme makes creating a menu, picking invitations, and designing the décor easier.

Baby shower themes should be lighthearted and silly, not serious or austere. This feeling will be conveyed in every detail from the invitation to the favor. Choosing a theme doesn't require that everything match exactly, but simply that details should coordinate and complement each other. The theme can be based on a color, a song title, a favorite hobby, or a gift idea. It can be as subtle and soft as a lullaby or as vibrant and edgy as rock and roll. It can, but does not have to, revolve entirely around the obvious topic of babies. There is only one rule: Make it fun—for you, the guests, and the guest of honor.

Factors to Consider Before Choosing a Theme

Theming a party can make it easier to plan; it provides an obvious path to decisions regarding invitation logos, napkin colors, cake motifs, centerpieces, and favors. Some themes lend themselves to specific activities, like a bowling party, or definitive décor, such as a Hawaiian luau theme. Some locations, like a fancy hotel, can accommodate a grandiose theme, while other venues, such as your home or backyard, require simplicity. Then, of course, there are certain locations that can only handle a hint of a theme, like restaurants and most work spaces.

Theme Considerations

There are some factors to consider when picking a shower theme. They are: the creative capabilities of the hostess (or cohostesses), any setup and cleanup issues, and time considerations.

✓ **Creative capabilities.** As the hostess, you will be handling the lion's share of the planning and preparing for the shower. Know your party-planning strengths and weaknesses. If you enjoy flexing your creativity, start with an imaginative and inventive theme and run with it! If, on the other hand, the thought of brainstorming a theme and gluing glitter on an invitation gives you a migraine—stop the madness! This is not a creativity contest. Open to the fast and fun theme chapters (Chapters 9–18) and pick a party that suits your fancy. Then apply lipstick, make a list of what you need, and get shopping.

✓ **Setup and cleanup issues.** Keep the theme in harmony with the environment. Wherever you plan to have the shower, think about what will be required to set up your theme and clean up the mess. Yes, it would be lovely to create a tropical paradise on the beach for your Barefoot and Pregnant Spa Shower, but five tons of sand in your mom's backyard might prove to be problematic at cleanup time. Avoid themes that will require architectural restructuring or excessive sweating and schlepping in your party clothes.

✓ **Time considerations.** The more elaborate the theme, the more time consuming its preparation. Do you have enough lead time? Can the shower location accommodate the time needed for setup and cleanup? If you are staging a shower at your workplace, you may only have forty-five minutes to an hour from start to finish. Don't decorate, celebrate!

Brainstorming the Shower Theme

Turning an idea into an event requires a brainstorming session. You can do it alone, but it is better to flex your creativity in a group. If you have cohosts, this is the perfect opportunity to meet and discuss party ideas. If you are planning a shower by yourself, don't worry, everybody has a little party planner in them; enlist your spouse, children, or other family members in the fun.

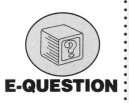

E-QUESTION

How do I kick off the planning party?

Whip up a pitcher of sangria and theme away. Take 2 bottles of red wine, 2 tablespoons of sugar, 2 ounces of brandy, 1 cup of orange juice, ½ a cup each of lemonade and limeade, and 1 orange, lemon, and lime, sliced into thin wheels. Combine ingredients. Store in the refrigerator until ready to serve. Add additional fruit to garnish. Serve in a pitcher or punch bowl.

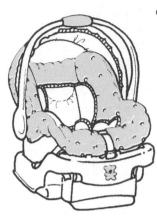

The very best way to brainstorm is to get your fellow cohostesses together with some refreshments, perhaps a good sangria recipe and some chips and salsa, and make it a party of its own.

This gathering shouldn't be complicated—in fact, to get the most out of the session, relaxation and fun need to be on the agenda. It also is helpful if you have blank paper (white boards, blackboards, etch-a-sketches, cocktail napkins, or doodle pads will also work), this book (naturally), and some spunky music in the background. You should also gather some style, home, baby, or entertaining magazines, and perhaps access to the Internet. The purpose of this "theming" get-together is to get the cohosts excited about the shower, to get the creative juices flowing, and to divvy up the workload. Ask a cohost to bring salsa and blue and yellow corn tortilla chips to go with your pitcher of sangria.

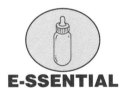

E-SSENTIAL

This Screamin' Themin' salsa will jump start your party planning. You will need 4 large tomatoes, seeded and diced; 2 small onions, finely chopped; one or two jalapeño peppers, finely chopped; 1 teaspoon of fresh-squeezed lime juice; 1 large bunch of cilantro leaves, cleaned and roughly chopped; and salt and freshly ground black pepper to taste. Toss together ingredients and serve with chips.

The Theme-Idea Worksheet in Appendix C will assist you and your shower cohosts in developing ideas that are tossed around the table. Give everyone a worksheet and a few minutes to jot down some thoughts, then open the floor for discussion and let the ideas fly. Sometimes what seems like a great idea is too difficult to translate into the shower details. Jot ideas and track how they morph into details on the worksheet.

Turning Simple Ideas into Great Themes

The great news about choosing a baby shower theme is that you don't have to go far for inspiration. Babies are so darn cute and they need everything, and so do new moms. You can build a theme around virtually anything. Go hunting for inspiration at a baby boutique, a stationery store, the mall, or even your grocery store. Search through your own closets and cupboards— are you inspired by a color, a dish pattern, a collection of teacups, floral sheets, or antique dolls? Use the list below for some shower theme ideas or to develop your own unusual shower themes:

- ✓ **Baby Gender:** Sugar and Spice, Little Princess, or Belles and Bows for a girl, and Snails and Puppy Dog Tails, Baby on Board, or Little Boy Blue if it's a boy
- ✓ **Babies in Groups:** Twins, triplets, and other multiples can be a theme of their own—Tea for Two, Peas in a Pod, Double Trouble
- ✓ **Baby's Layette:** Booties, onesies, drawstring night sacs, and bonnets
- ✓ **Baby's Nursery:** Carriages, cribs, bottles, diaper pins, and pacifiers
- ✓ **Baby's Toys:** Ducks, bunnies, lambs, giraffes, elephants, rattles, teddy bears, trucks, trains, dolls, and blocks
- ✓ **Baby Animals:** Puppies, chicks, kittens, birds
- ✓ **Baby's Schedule:** Feeding time, bath time, naptime, bedtime
- ✓ **Baby Icons:** Hearts, flowers, angels, clouds, rainbows, bows, buttons, stork
- ✓ **Nursery Rhymes, Lullabies, and Literature:** "The Cow Jumped Over the Moon," *Good Night Moon,* "Cat and the Fiddle," Dr. Seuss, *The Tale of Peter Rabbit,* "Twinkle, Twinkle Little Star"
- ✓ **Seasonal Themes:** Christmas, Hanukkah, Valentine's Day, Fourth of July, Thanksgiving, Halloween, winter, spring, summer, or fall
- ✓ **Colors and Patterns:** Pastels, primary, monochromatic, nursery colors, pink, blue, yellow, green, lavender; patterns like checks, polka dots, and stripes
- ✓ **Flowers:** Sunflowers, tulips, roses, baby's breath, violets, pansies, daisies

✓ **Guest Demographics:** Mommy's girlfriends, coworkers, Grandmother's friends, cousins, couples, neighbors, book club, religious community, bowling league, etc.

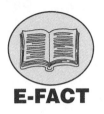

E-FACT

Most men will put on the brakes at the idea of a party with tea sandwiches, baby clothes, or shower games. Go with a guy-centric (but mommy-safe) theme from this book, an interesting activity, and a hearty menu served up with a microbrew, and you will have the male contingent cheering.

Themes from Movies, Television, and Pop Culture

Movies, television, and pop culture offer a treasure-trove of ideas. There are theme "jewels" to be found, but you may need to stretch your imagination and give a potential idea a bit of a twist to make it work for baby. The results can be unconventional, but that may suit your style. One thing is certain: It will give your shower a personality all its own.

Some entertainment-inspired shower ideas include:

✓ **A "Survivor" Shower.** If you have a fun-loving set of parents-to-be who are *Survivor* groupies, you could turn this interest into a great theme with a built-in activity—a Survivor-esque baby-care competition: Survivor: the Nursery Edition—Out Bathe, Out Diaper, Out Burp. An afternoon of barbequing complete with palm trees, s'mores, and a tribal council to decide who will survive the nursery challenge and who will be voted off the island.

✓ **An American Lullaby Idol Shower.** This star-studded theme opportunity starts with a star-struck invitation for couples. Let guests know that they will be competing for the coveted title of American Lullaby Idol. Karaoke is the activity d'jour—menu options could include a make-your-own panini bar and brownies with peanut butter ice cream. Set up a shimmer curtain to create a "stage" and set the mood to shine. Award extra points for creating your own lullaby lyrics. Winner takes home a trophy and bragging rights.

✓ **A Superbawl Sunday Shower.** This may be the easiest way to have a couples shower, especially during football season. Gather friends on any Sunday, kick off with beer and chili dogs, add baby gifts and a due-date pool, and you've got a touchdown!

✓ **A Diapering with the Stars Shower.** Get moving! A local dance club or bar may be the perfect setting for dancing and diapering. Create a Diapering Line Dance or the Boot-Scooting Baby Boogie. Tell guests to wear something pink or blue, if you know the baby's gender. Then get ready to boogie down.

Or perhaps you like the concept of the TV/movie shower theme, but still want something different? Start by making a list of favorite movies, television shows, or pop-culture icons. Then play around with the words, sounds, and letters. Try adding a baby item to replace a word in a title—as in Drool or No Drool (borrowed from the television show *Deal or No Deal*). Another way to come up with a theme is to start with a phrase; "Cute as a Button" or "Boys will be Boys," both of which would work well as shower themes and can easily be carried through every detail.

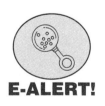

E-ALERT!

A unique shower theme can present a décor and invitation challenge. A plethora of preprinted and prepackaged supplies for classically themed showers—like Winnie-the-Pooh—are readily available. Not so for some of the more unusual themes. If you love the creative process, you'll rise to the challenge; however, if time (and creativity) is short, opt for a more traditional theme.

Fashionable Themes

Capturing a current fashion trend is another way to create an up-to-the-minute baby shower theme. For the mother-to-be who is a trend-setter herself, this method will be a match made in Hollywood. Creating a theme based on fashion is as easy as a trip to the video store. *The Devil Wears Prada* quickly becomes The Devil Wears Diapers. Trends in fashion can be a cache of ideas for the shower-throwing chic. Watch the Style network and peruse fashion magazines for the pivotal piece of inspiration. Here are some ideas for the fashion-themed shower:

- ✓ **The Thoroughly Modern Mamma Shower.** The invitations feature a belly-bursting fashionista ready to take on life and baby couture. Choose bold patterns and colors and mix it up with black, aluminum, or stainless steel for a contemporary edge. Décor is all about repeated pattern against a minimal backdrop of white or black. Keep the lines clean—centerpieces can consist of a row of single Gerber daisies in small square vases interspersed with martini glasses filled with white jelly beans. An Asian chicken salad, Sour Apple "mocktini," and wontons with chocolate dipping compliment this modern theme.

- ✓ **The Project Bellybump Shower.** Take a cue from *Project Runway* for a shower with a fashion challenge: Bringing up baby with a strong sense of fashion! Project Bellybump: A Baby Shoe-er is a call for baby shoes—fun, fabulous, and fashionable! Project Bellybump: Recycled! offers a fashion booster shot for mommy-to-be's maternity wardrobe. Guests are encouraged to give fashion accessories, recycled maternity wear, or trendy baby clothes.

  The shower concept is fashion forward and fun. Use bracelets for napkin rings; drape a chandelier with pearl necklaces. Keep the menu simple—serve wine (alcoholic and nonalcoholic) and cheese. Fashion magazines can play two roles, décor and favors.

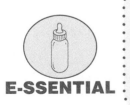

E-SSENTIAL

Hobbies, special interests, and specific locations are also sources for a terrific theme. If the parents-to-be are avid bocce ball players, bowlers, or golfers, you can use this interest to spark some theme ideas. Knitting, crafting, rowing, cooking—these hobbies can also prompt a slew of shower ideas.

Gifts That Inspire Themes

Gifts can deliver more than a present—they can become the inspiration for a fantastic shower concept. Using a specific category of gift to theme your shower is great if the soon-to-be-mommy is having more than one shower. Focus on a single category of present—layette, bath time, travel needs, equipment, meal time, or even just diapers. Then build the theme around this gift group. Some ideas for gift-inspired showers could include:

- ✓ **Splish-Splash—Baby Needs a Bath.** Gifts of bath-time supplies from lotion to tub toys can be the beginning of a squeaky-clean theme. Carry out this theme with a rubber ducky on the invitation and a row of them down the table center. Decorate with bright yellow and punches of blue (for a boy) or hot pink (for a girl). Consider using terry washcloths as napkins and giving bath-soap favors, tied with a yellow ribbon and embellished with a giant diaper pin.

- ✓ **Shake, Rattle, and Roll: A Shower for a Baby Born to Travel.** If the family-to-be has a penchant for travel, this is the shower for them. Tie a colorful rattle with a shipping-tag invitation and ask guests to give a gift for the traveling baby; such as car toys, a sand stroller, a travel bed, a beach tent, or a baby-sling carrier. Bento-box lunches are portable, interesting, and offer an international flavor to the festivities. A mini-suitcase centerpiece explodes with packable baby necessities—wipes, suntan lotion, disposable bibs, and the like. Give the new parents a stack of preaddressed postcards and a digital camera to capture precious moments. This party can be tweaked to be trip specific—right down to the gifts—camping gear, beach-friendly equipment, or overseas travel needs. So get ready to get these new parents ready to roll.

- ✓ **Calendar Kid: Baby Needs Month-by-Month.** They are little, but their needs change with every passing day. Assign guests a month or a range of months and ask them to bring something that baby would need or enjoy in that developmental period. Make sure you put the due date on the invitation to assist guests in choosing their gift. Invitations could look like a calendar page. Create a centerpiece that Mommy can take home—twelve matching picture frames to display baby each month for the first year. Fill frames with baby facts for each month. Incorporate the calendar theme into a game or activity. Mini calendars can be custom ordered and make useful shower favors.

Going Themeless

Some showers are better left themeless. In fact, it's a bit of a trend. With modern life so wrapped in chaos, there is a minimalist trend in party giving that extends to baby showers as well. People still want to offer "congrats" on the upcoming arrival of baby, but they also like an excuse to host a pared-down party. These modern baby showers feel more like regular parties with the addition of presents rather than traditional baby showers. Whether you decide to host a couple's cocktail party or a girls' night out, going themeless is another alternative for today's über-chic baby showers.

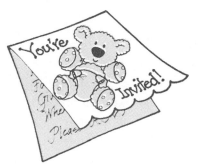

Chapter 4

Invitations

NOTHING IS A BETTER showcase for inspiration than the spokesperson for your party: the invitation. It is a welcoming indication that a party is on the way. The best thing about a baby shower invitation is that it can scream with joy and burst with exuberant color. It is a no-holds-barred "Come on in" to family, friends, and mommy-to-be. Whether your invitation is store-bought, handcrafted, computer-generated, e-mailed, or custom-printed, it will announce the happy occasion. With the many options available today, choosing and creating the invitations can be one of the most enjoyable parts of putting the shower together.

Who to Invite

You (and your cohosts) have chosen a theme, venue, and basic guest count for your party. Now it's time finalize the guest list and gather the most current names and addresses. Communication is very important at this stage in the planning. A call to the mommy-to-be is the first order of business. Be very specific about the parameters of the party you are proposing. Tell her where the shower will be held and what the space or monetary restrictions may be. Let her know how many people you can accommodate and ask her to give you a list of names with that number plus a few extras. If it is a surprise shower, a call to the husband, best friend, or mother may be in order, to gather the particulars of the guest list. Remember that it's better to invite too many people and risk being crowded than to overlook some people and hurt their feelings.

Some showers have ready-made guest lists; for example, if the book club is throwing a shower, the guest list will be limited to club members. There's nothing wrong with that. Babies (and mommies) can't be showered with too much love. It's always a nice touch to invite the girl's mother, mother-in-law, or husband, but again, it is not mandatory or necessary to include them if the group throwing the shower is not a part of their social circle.

How to Invite

It seems that in today's modern culture there is no end to the number of ways we can invite others to a party. Although a shower is the type of party that can be handled with a phone call or note, there is something nice about receiving a written invitation, preferably one that is fun and interesting. Even if you have two left feet when it comes to making things, you will find that it is not the complexity of the invite but the sense of party that it conveys that will leave the most favorable impression.

✓ **Handwritten invitations.** A handwritten note is a time-honored method of inviting people to a shower. In fact, it stands out in the sea of computer-generated clip art invites you have become accustomed to receiving. Choose a good quality stationery, use a comfortable pen (gel pens have a good flow and come in many attractive colors), and after a practice run, put your best penmanship to work. This option is perfect for a small shower with fifteen invitations or less.

✓ **Preprinted invitations.** These invitations can be located at a variety of places, including your local stationery or card shop, many drugstores, or party stores. These invitations typically feature some cute artwork on the front and have fill-in lines for your party information on the inside. There are lots of options available on the Web for this type of invitation as well. This is an excellent option for any shower.

✓ **Handmade invitations.** Here's where the creative juices start to flow. If you feel comfortable with crafts, or have some computer knowledge, these invitations can be made easily and offer a huge variety of designs.

✓ **Custom printed invitations.** Card shops, such as Hallmark, Papyrus, and the like, can use preprinted designs to custom print your invitations. Of course, you can also take your project to a local printer, but the cost of small-run printing jobs can be exorbitant.

✓ **Electronic invitations.** Evite.com is one of many one-stop online invitation- and party-design Web sites that offers electronic invitations. You can choose a design, type in all the information, and with the push of a button your invitations are created and mailed. You can track R.S.V.P.s online, and send nonresponsive guests an e-mail reminder to respond. This is a perfect invitation for workplace parties or if the group to be invited is "well connected." The downside to this form of invitation is that not all your guests may have access to e-mail. In addition, there is no physical invitation to thumbtack to a bulletin board or hang on your refrigerator.

What to Include on the Invitation

The prime purpose of the invitation is to impart critical information about your shower to the people you want to come. Even if the party is a surprise to the mother-to-be, do not try to surprise the guests. The invitation should also convey the spirit of the shower. A whimsical phrase or quote or a clever turn of phrase that incorporates your theme helps to set the tone for the happy time to come.

People want and need to know what to expect—whether it's dinner or lunch or a snack—what to bring, what to wear, how fancy or casual the party will be, and any other particulars that will affect the guests. It's the hostess's job to prepare the guests for the event, and it's the invitation's job to deliver that information. Here's what every invitation should include:

- ✓ Date, time, and length of the shower (i.e., when you want them to arrive and leave)
- ✓ Who is included in the invitation (kids, dogs, spouses or mates)
- ✓ The name of the mother-to-be and the baby's name and/or gender if known in advance
- ✓ A map to your house or the location (if specific information is needed to get there)
- ✓ Gift information (the registry, themed gift ideas like the layette shower, etc.)
- ✓ Meal to be included (If you are serving a meal, mention dinner and drinks, a luncheon, a brunch, cocktails and appetizers, etc.)
- ✓ What to wear, if necessary (e.g., "Everyone should wear something pink," or "swimsuits and jeans," etc.)
- ✓ R.S.V.P. information—such as a phone number or e-mail address (essential if you need a food count)
- ✓ A deadline to respond to the R.S.V.P.

Handling the R.S.V.P.s

Party responses come in waves. One or two guests will call you so quickly that you wonder if the guest was clairvoyant. Others trickle in as the deadline approaches. And some guests simply call at the very, very last minute or neglect to call at all. Most party planners agree that for every twenty to twenty-five guests you invite, three to five won't attend. If you haven't heard from a potential guest, it is acceptable to give them a call to verify they have received the invitation. The issue of responses can be tricky, and many hostesses have been undone worrying that their occasion will be ruined by no-shows. Remember this: The people who want to be there and should be there will be there, and the party will be great with the guests that are there.

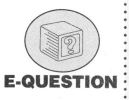

What does R·S·V·P· mean?

R.S.V.P. is an acronym for the French phrase *Répondez, s'il vous plaît*, which means, "please, respond." French hostesses got tired of not knowing at the last minute who was coming and how many to set for dinner. It made party throwing so much easier that people have been using it ever since.

To track responses, generate a list of those you invited. If you have given a phone number to respond to, keep the list near the phone so you have easy access as your guests call to say yes to the shower. You may also want to keep any pertinent information or updates nearby as well, in case curious guests ask the baby's gender, or special needs, or whether Auntie Sue is coming. Be sure to let your family know that you are expecting calls. Tell them how you wish for them to handle taking information down.

Creative Ideas for Invitations

There are a number of avenues you can explore when creating your perfect invitation. They are the use of color, use of pattern, addition of layers, use of fonts as design, and the use of multiple materials. So take your theme for a test drive with some of these invitation jump-start ideas. Your destination is an invitation that will give your guests a glimpse of the party to come.

Using Color

Colors can be dramatic, subtle, electrifying, calming, sweet, or bold—they set the tone for your event, and there are endless combination possibilities. Here are some ideas for incorporating color in your invitation design.

✓ **Single color.** A single color, used with white or black, is a simple, but highly effective, design choice. Pale pink polka dots or stripes can set a clean, crisp, and happy tone to welcome a baby girl. Turn up the volume to hot pink and sweet becomes trendy. Pale yellow is pretty, but a bright yellow chick cut out of cardstock is bold and modern.

✓ **Multiple colors.** The showers your mother attended invariably featured pastels on parade. Ducks, bunnies, bears, and lambs in soft hues were the icons du jour that marched across most invitations. While pastels are always available, current moms-to-be favor trendier palettes: robin's-egg blue with milk chocolate, turquoise and mandarin orange, sparkling lime and lavender are just a few of today's modern color combinations.

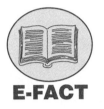

E-FACT

According to Michelle Martin of Out of the Envelope, an invitation specialty shop in Los Gatos, California, baby shower invitations can be as low as $1 each but can run as high as $10 each for custom-printed or embellished designs. Extras like gluing, coloring, glittering, beribboning, and hand addressing can push up the total cost of any invitation.

Using Fonts

Words can become an element of invitation design. By choosing a special font, you can easily create great design without using clip art, drawings, or pictures. There are thousands of font styles available today. Most word-processing software comes with some great fonts as a standard part of the package. You can also purchase fonts from the Web or packaged as add-ons for use with a particular software program. Some Web sites offer free fonts, which are available for download directly to your computer (as with all downloads, please practice good Web security). The ideas for font usage given here will require the use of a computer and word-processing software. If you are technology-challenged, your local invitation store can help you work with fonts.

Fonts are offered in a variety of sizes, called points. The font called Times New Roman in 12-point format is the default font for most word-processing programs. A 6-point font is tiny, usually found on business cards. A 72-point font is quite large. For invitations, typically a 10- to 12-point font is fine for general information, and you can embellish or emphasize with font sizes ranging from 20 to 30 points.

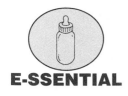

E-SSENTIAL

These fonts can convey a girlier tone when a baby girl is the guest of honor: *Viner Hand, Amazone TC, Caliban,* and ChildSplay. When planning a shower for a boy, consider these fonts instead of the traditional ones: Copperplate Gothic, **Postino**, Binner Gothic, or **Ad Lib.**

When using fonts, keep these tips in mind:

✓ **Vary font size:** Emphasize key words or phrases in a larger font size. For added emphasis, outline them or use the "bold" command on your word-processing software.

✓ **Vary font style:** Fonts are fun. Play around with different styles. Highlight key words or names in a fancy font, like Nuptials or Zapf Chancery, then leave the rest in a simple font, such as Arial or Century Gothic. Although it is possible to use a different font on every word, it can be difficult to read. Two to three font styles can give you an interesting look without creating chaos.

✓ **Vary font colors:** Try highlighting certain key words in a theme color. "A Shower for Kerry" could be in hot pink, with the balance of words in gray, black, or brown.

Using Pattern

Pattern—the repeat of shapes, lines, and colors—can be an important element in invitation design. Patterned paper can be used in touches or as the backdrop for an entire invitation; it can also be used to line an envelope. You can create patterns with cutouts, rubber stamps, stickers, and pens, to name a few.

To create a single-element pattern you can feature one large shape, such as a baby bottle, in your design or reduce its size and repeat it all over the invitation in a random or organized arrangement. Cupcakes, hearts, booties, rattles, diaper pins, baby buggies, and baby T-shirts can all be used to create a design.

For our overachievers, try creating a design with more than one element; alternating hearts and rattles, roses and pacifiers, or any other combination. You can also have random patterns—in this case, try overlapping some of the elements to create a cohesive look.

Adding Materials and Layers

Here's the fun stuff! You've chosen a color scheme. You've thought about a pattern or design element. Adding materials and layers to an invitation has the same effect as accessorizing an outfit. It adds interest and pizzazz to your look and gives it the perfect finishing touch.

As with fashion accessories, you can go overboard. So start with your basic invitation and build it up slowly: For example, you want to include pink polka dots in your basic design. Use plain white paper for the wording, a pink polka-dot paper as a border, and hot-pink cardstock for a background. Then glue several hot-pink buttons in the corners and you've got a party invitation.

E-FACT

Many art and craft stores carry specialty papers that you won't find anywhere else. You can add a strip of paper or a whole sheet, depending on the look you want to create. Colored cardstock (matte or glossy), rice paper, gift wrap, origami paper, handmade paper with herbs or flowers, or recycled, vellum, parchment, gold-flecked, metallic, or antiqued papers are all possibilities.

You can incorporate vintage postcards, old photos, shipping tags, ring tags, even holiday cards into your invitation design. Any specialty paper can become a layer on your creation.

Once you have built up the flat layers, you are ready to add a dimensional element to finish your project. As mentioned above, buttons will work, but you can also use ribbon, yarn, rhinestones, glitter, rickrack, lace, stickers, beads, and charms.

Personalizing Store-Bought Invitations

Many drug stores, stationery stores, and the like offer a selection of simple but effective invitation designs that will be perfect for your event. If you've fallen in love with an adorable invitation from the local paper store, but you want to spruce it up a little bit, here are some ideas:

✓ **Glitter.** Glitter glues and pens can add a dot or line of sparkle and make any invite shine.

✓ **Bejewel.** Nothing can beat the effect of a well-placed rhinestone or other "jewel." Pearls, beads, or gems will dress up bonnets, booties, and baby carriages that are featured in many of the current invitation designs.

✓ **Stickers.** Stickers now come in fabulous designs. You can get a roll of black stilettos as well as the more traditional chicks and ducks that frequent many baby shower invites.

✓ **Scissors.** A new breed of scissors has emerged that will give your invitations a fancy edge. In addition to the classic zig-zag scissors (known as pinking shears), you can now find scissors that create a "deckled" edge, scalloped edge, spiked edge, or wavy edge. Your local craft or office-supply store will carry these or others.

Designing Handmade Invitations

A terrific resource for creating an invitation from scratch is your local scrap-booking store. They specialize in the bows and furbelows that are the perfect scale for any type of invitation. They also carry rubber stamps, colored and metallic inks, specialty papers, and loads of ideas that will feed your creativity and carry forward your theme ideas with élan.

Out-of-the-Ordinary Invitations

If you feel that the occasion you are planning needs an extra-special invite, and if your budget allows it, you can go all out. Invitations don't have to be flat or arrive in an envelope. They can be delivered by a stork (husbands make excellent storks!) or come in a fancy box. They can even taste good!

The baby-bottle invitation is an example of an over-the-top invite. Like a modern-day message in a bottle, a baby bottle filled with jellybeans and the party's vital statistics will pack a punch when received by your guests. You can mail these in one of two ways: Add a mailing label and the correct postage and send them "naked" or put them in a mailing tube (available at most packaging stores), and off they go.

For those moms-to-be with a sweet tooth, the candy box invitation is another great way to say "Please come." A 5" × 5" cardboard jewelry box is the starting point for these yummy invites. Party information is printed on cardstock and placed in the box cover, and in the box, a candy necklace or other candy favorite is revealed. You can make this yourself or order them online at *www.plumparty.com*.

E-FACT

The United States Postal Service has a great way to calculate postage—the Web. Simply go to *www.usps.gov* and click the "Calculate Postage" tab. You can enter the type of mailing (postcard, envelope, etc.) and the "to" and "from" zip codes. You're two clicks away from the exact postage needed for your invitations.

Special Delivery Options for Invitations

Once you have decorated, printed, colored, or rubber-stamped your invitations, they will need to be posted. An oversized invitation is always interesting, but it can double or triple the cost of postage. In addition, adding buttons, diaper pins, and other accoutrements can add weight and may require larger envelopes. This also adds additional expense. The post office has mailing and packaging information on its Web site, or you can go into any branch and have them weigh a mock-up invitation.

Be sure to mail the invitations four to six weeks before your shower date. If you are inviting people from out of town to the shower, remember that airline reservations are much, much cheaper if they are made at least thirty days in advance, so work that into your invitation mailing schedule.

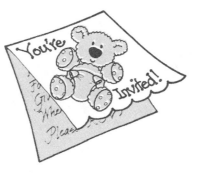

Chapter 5

The Art and Science of Menu Selection

THE PREPARATION OF DELICIOUS, beautifully presented food is an art, but there is a science to selecting the menu. Shower menus can run the gamut from cake and ice cream to cocktails and appetizers and from tea and biscuits to a five-course gourmet dinner. Now it is time to apply some common sense to the science of the menu selection and food preparation. This chapter will help you choose a menu that is delicious and comfortable for the way you like to entertain.

Menu Basics

As you begin the menu selection process, you will need to take into consideration the following:

- ✓ The shower theme
- ✓ Layout of the shower venue
- ✓ The style of the shower
- ✓ The time of day (breakfast, brunch, lunch, cocktails, dinner, or après-dinner)
- ✓ The time of year (spring, summer, fall, winter)
- ✓ The number of guests
- ✓ Who will be handling the food preparation

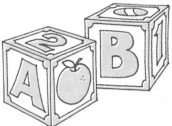

Seating, Serving, and Style

Your shower food should fit your shower style. A formal shower calls for formal food—china and caviar at a barbeque just doesn't work. Find the best way to serve up the best food with the least amount of stress to you, the hostess, whether that means baking ahead, buying in bulk, ordering out, or catering in. The only rule about doing it right is making it comfortable for everybody.

Method of Food Service

The method you choose to serve the food will play an important role in the menu you select. A formal dinner requires that guests be seated and that food is served on a proper dinner plate with proper flatware. Inventory your supplies to see how many plates, glasses, and serving pieces you have. Will it be enough for the number of people you are inviting? If not, how will you make up the difference? You could rent what you need or you may decide to go casual and use paper goods. With a casual setting and theme, a plate of "small bites," held on a lap or perched on a cocktail table, is perfectly acceptable. Here are the three types of food service:

✓ **Passed service.** Frequently seen at cocktail parties, this type of food service requires staff devoted to going guest to guest with trays of appetizers and drinks. Those manning the serving trays should be adept at juggling a tray of drinks and a handful of cocktail napkins. If this is the service style you have chosen, consider hiring professional waitstaff.

✓ **Self-service.** The buffet is the most common way to serve food to a crowd. It allows the food to be arranged on a serving table, and then guests go to the table, take utensils and a plate, and serve themselves. It works well in most homes and with most age groups. It also requires fewer people to manage the food service. You can use paper plates, paper napkins, and plastic forks or china, cloth napkins, and silverware for a buffet.

✓ **Plated service.** This style of service can be dressed up or dressed down. Obviously, it requires table-and-chair seating for all the guests. This is perfect for groups of ten or less. Even if your home can accommodate a larger group, a sit-down meal may require an extra set of hands (or two) to serve everyone.

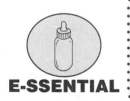

E-SSENTIAL

For the home buffet, a five- to six-foot table is the minimum requirement for setting up food, plates, and dining accoutrements. Use the extension leaves on your dining room or kitchen table, or bring in a six-foot folding table. If you are covering the buffet table with a cloth, choosing floor-length linens makes a better presentation.

Food Trafficking

Those in the food-service industry know that as soon as the first tray of food is set on the serving table, a buffet line will form instantaneously. And as the hostess, that's when you'll be glad you considered this issue of food and traffic. If you are hosting the shower in a home, look at doorways and hallways in relation to the placement of the buffet table. If you do not want guests to sit at the buffet table, remove the chairs and place them elsewhere in the room.

Set up the table to allow traffic to flow on all sides, rather than just one side. Place plates, napkins, and utensils together at the starting point of the buffet line. Allow space at the edge of the table for guests to rest a plate as they serve themselves. When hosting a large group, have two sets of food and place one on each side of the table—two bowls of the salad, two trays of the chicken, and so on, to ease congestion. If your group is more than twenty, set up two buffet tables or consider food stations around the room or in other rooms of your home. Set up a beverage area away from the food table, which will also prevent a bottleneck as the food is served.

Sitting Pretty

Menu faux pas can be avoided during the planning, but they are hard to correct at the shower! Nothing is more embarrassing than to arrive at a party all dressed up, sit down at the edge of a chintz-covered couch, and spill a droopy paper plate filled with barbequed beast all down the front of your outfit and the couch. It's also embarrassing to be introduced to the mother of the guest of honor with a chicken wing in your hand. Food that is too spicy, too saucy, too drippy, too sticky, too crumbly, and too hard to eat is not a great idea for a ladies tea, but may be perfect for a backyard barbeque shower with family.

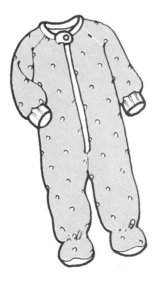

Basic Food Rules

Although this book advocates a creative approach to most things culinary, there are still some rules for parties. Selecting a menu takes consideration, creativity, and some calculations. If you are an adventurous chef, this is not the time to try out a new recipe or challenge guests with "Guess what we ate for dinner?" Instead, it is a time to exercise your serving creativity on tried-and-true recipes that you know to be crowd pleasers. It is not the time to choose a meal that requires a week off to prepare and a week's vacation to recover from preparing.

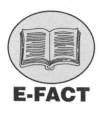

E-FACT

Some foods are not recommended for pregnant women. These include sushi, deep-sea fish (high in mercury), unpasteurized cheeses and dairy products, undercooked meats, and foods laden with sodium. Excessive caffeine and alcohol are also not recommended, so watch when considering these menu items.

Name That Meal

The time of day generally dictates the type of meal you will serve. Traditionally, the shower is held around lunch; however, today's showers can be held at any time. Each meal has some basic elements that you must keep in mind as you select the shower menu.

Breakfast

Served until 11:00 A.M., breakfast comes in two styles: full and continental. A full breakfast includes eggs and breakfast meats like sausage, bacon, or ham. Pastries, toast, potatoes, and vegetables (e.g., asparagus spears) along with coffee and tea are all customary components of the full breakfast. A continental breakfast consists of baked goods like muffins, croissants, scones, and nut breads, along with an assortment of juices, coffee, and tea.

For a simple buffet breakfast, you should have:

✓ Eggs—scrambled or poached hold up best
✓ Bacon, sausage, or ham
✓ Two types of baked goods (e.g., scones and blueberry muffins)
✓ Coffee—decaffeinated and regular
✓ Tea—herbal and green or black
✓ Variation: Add French toast as a second main dish and a "mamatini mocktail" (see page 50)

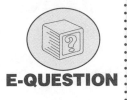

What's a mocktail?
Mocktails are cocktails without the alcohol. A Mamatini, perfect for the mother-to-be, is a breakfast martini. Mocktail: 1½ ounces gingerale, ¾ ounce fresh lemon juice, ¾ ounce orange juice, 1 teaspoon marmalade. Garnish with orange peel and serve in a martini glass.

Brunch

Served from 10:00 A.M. to 2:00 P.M., a brunch is a combination of breakfast and lunch. Brunches are usually held on a weekend day. You can usually find eggs on the menu, but they are in the form of a quiche or in a crepe. A refreshing salad and assortments of rolls, cheeses, and fruits are also common. A brunch-menu buffet should include at least one breakfast entrée, such as eggs Benedict, quiche, or baked eggs; a lunch entrée, for example, spinach Florentine crepes; and one salad, like Asian chicken salad or a Cobb salad. There should be a dessert item as well, which could be simply a cake or tray of cookies. Champagne or mimosas (champagne and orange juice) and sparkling apple juice often accompany a brunch.

Lunch

Served from 11:30 A.M. to 2:00 P.M., the difference between brunch and lunch is the food served, not the time it is served. Guests invited to a luncheon shower would expect a main-course salad, sandwich, or entrée rather than egg dishes. A plated lunch at a restaurant may include soup, salad, and a hot or cold entrée, as well as dessert. If you are hosting at home, a single entrée or main course salad with bread followed by the dessert is perfectly acceptable. If the guest list is all women, a Caesar salad with poached chicken is fine, but if men will be attending, select a heartier meal or add a sandwich to the fare.

Tea (Traditional English)

Tea is served from 3:00 P.M. to 6:00 P.M. Afternoon tea is served until 5:00 P.M., while high tea, which is more like a light dinner, is served between

5:00 P.M. and 6:00 P.M. Teas, whether in the early or late afternoon, consist of a menu ranging from scones, jams, and tarts to savory sandwiches of egg salad, tuna salad, or cucumber and watercress, finishing with an array of tiny and tempting dessert pastries. Usually two to four different types of tea are offered in the traditional English tea service.

Cocktails

Cocktails are served from 4:00 P.M. to 7:00 P.M. (also called happy hour) or 6:00 P.M. to 9:00 P.M. A cocktail party covers a wide range of menu options. "Happy Hour" implies that there will be some food and alcoholic beverages but not necessarily dinner. Salty snacks, such as pretzels, nuts, and chips, and appetizers such as crudités or mini-quesadillas or pizzas make up the menu. A classic cocktail party features a more robust menu designed to allow guests to move freely and mingle. Food should be bite-sized, plentiful, and portable. A full bar is not necessary; plan on serving one or two signature drinks, such as mojitos and pink or blue cosmopolitans. A full stomach is a must—so plan on generous servings of everything edible. Cocktail fare can be simple, but variety is important. Consider serving four to six types of appetizers and something sweet for dessert.

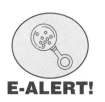

E-ALERT!

People come to cocktail parties hungry! Figure on four to six appetizer pieces per person per hour, especially if you will not be serving dinner. Always include a meat option and a vegetarian option, and don't be surprised if people go crazy for the meat—it's filling and tempting in tiny bites.

Dinner

Dinner parties start from 5:00 P.M. to 8:00 P.M. Any party in this time frame that doesn't specify otherwise brings with it the expectation of dinner. Plated dinners usually feature meat or poultry; a vegetable or salad; and potatoes, rice, or pasta. If you are sitting at a table, food can be preplated or served family style. Dessert can be served at the table or in another room shortly after the dinner is over. For a buffet, two entrées, a salad or pasta, bread, and dessert are fine.

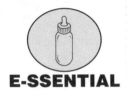

E-SSENTIAL

To keep the buffet line moving and reduce food questions, label each dish with the name and main ingredients. A menu card can be created on your computer or can be handwritten. Consider giving the dish a name that not only describes it but also works with the shower theme; for example, Baby Carriage Cacciatore with chicken, basil, and sausage.

Just Desserts

Desserts can be served in the afternoon, evening, or at break time during a workday. Specify on the invitation that it's dessert only. Cake is the traditional shower dessert. You can serve it plain or with ice cream. If you want to amp up the menu a bit, consider a dessert bar or buffet. A dessert bar uses one dessert—say cupcakes—then expands on that theme by offering multiple flavors or mix-and-match toppings, frost-your-own, and so on. A dessert buffet presents a variety of different desserts, such as cheesecake, brownies, a cookie tray, and rice pudding.

Food Rules

Now that you've decided when to serve (breakfast, lunch, dinner) and how to serve (buffet, sit-down, passed), you are at the point of deciding what to serve and how to present it. Food is a sensory experience—you smell it, see it, taste it, feel it's textures. It's a feast for the eyes and palette, even if you are serving just one dish.

As you start to create your menu, incorporate a sensory run-through. How will the plate look? Are the foods you are planning to serve of similar color and texture? Mashed potatoes, sliced turkey breast, and creamed onions are all delicious, but on the same plate they are visually boring. Green beans would be a great addition to this plate and this menu. Green beans with slivered almonds would be an even better choice. Plan your menu to include a variety of flavors, textures, and colors to create a menu that has visual and sensory appeal.

Food Variety and Texture

You do not need a wide variety of foods at a shower, but the foods you do choose should complement each other without being repetitive. Don't repeat a main ingredient in another dish. Creamed spinach, spinach salad, and chicken spinach casserole is spinach overload. Mix sweet flavors with savory ones, like pork chops and applesauce; balance hot flavors with cool, such as spicy chili with sour cream. Too many sauces, competing gravies, and too many rich foods are also not recommended.

The texture of foods is another way to expand the sensory experience and add variety to the menu. Crunchy salads are delicious with tender pasta dishes. Pignolis (pine nuts) offer a contrast to steamed vegetables. Crispy steak fries are the perfect companion to a great filet mignon.

Food Presentation

The way food is presented is an art form in and of itself. You do not need elaborate presentations, but you do need to think about how the food will look as it's presented on the plate. For most home showers, there will be a central food table set up for a buffet. The table will contain platters, bowls, and trays of the various foods prepared. To make your table visually appealing, consider the following:

✓ **Color.** A tray of tomatoes garnished with herbs, a platter of roasted chicken breast, and a bowl of salad with fresh peas, red peppers, and romaine lettuce will not only be yummy, but colorful and interesting as well.

✓ **Shape.** Use food shapes as a design element. Round, red new potatoes, narrow strips of yellow pepper, asparagus spears, carrots cut on the diagonal, melon balls, and pineapple chunks all bring an added level of visual excitement to your menu. Consider both natural shapes of foods as well as the shapes you can create with slicing and dicing.

✓ **Garnish.** The garnish is a food accessory. It finishes the presentation and creates a well-dressed plate. A handful of fresh herbs, a sprinkling of toasted sesame seeds, a swirl of crème fraîche, or a dusting of cocoa powder can be the finishing touch.

Hostess in Labor

The mother-to-be isn't the only one who will be in labor. As the hostess, you will be in labor, too—"party labor." Unlike the expectant mommy who doesn't yet know how long her labor will be, the hostess will be in labor for days, even weeks. The good news is that you can be in control of yours—with a little preplanning. As you read through the ideas in this book, remember to balance the details of the party the same way you balance the flavors in the recipes. If your party is heavy on the decorations, go light on the food preparations. A complicated menu may work best with a less involved theme. Don't discount the time and labor you will expend getting your house, your table, and yourself ready for your shindig.

✓ **Plan for prep time.** Choose recipes that can be prepared a day or two ahead. You cannot spend the day of the shower in the kitchen chopping, braising, or sautéing. The only kitchen activities should be heating, plattering, and garnishing. And you should enlist extra helping hands for last-minute food details. When guests arrive, you shouldn't be in the shower; you must be at the shower, in all your glory.

✓ **Serving temperature.** Choose foods that are delicious both hot and at room temperature. Salmon is the chef's choice at large functions because it maintains its flavor whether hot off the grill or cooled down. Avoid choosing foods that spoil easily, especially if your party is scheduled for a hot-weather season.

✓ **Plan for clean up.** When the party's over, the task of cleaning up can be daunting, particularly in the kitchen. Do yourself a favor and enlist some help, either volunteer or paid, to assist you in getting things back in order. When you are having a crowd, even one paid staffer will make an enormous difference.

✓ **Test the recipes.** Leave nothing to chance—test your recipes. Have a trial run (or two) on your family before you whip up something for a crowd. This will allow you to fine-tune the flavor, bone-up on the techniques, and work out the flaws in timing and serving. The run-through will also give you a chance to prepare mentally for the party.

E-SSENTIAL

If you are a co-hostess who has offered to bring a food item to the shower, come prepared by bringing your own food station! Bring EVERYTHING you will need to cut, slice, garnish, and present your offering, from paring knife to platter. Once it is ready to be served, pack up your equipment and supplies and move them out of sight. You will win the heart of the hostess.

Pack-and-Go Foods

There is no law that says the hostess must prepare all the food from scratch. There is also no prize to the hostess who does. So simplify whenever you can. Grocery stores now have a range of prepared dishes that are tasty, cost effective, and finished. From shrimp platters to deli trays, cookies, cakes, salads, and more—you can order everything ahead or supplement what you don't have the time or inclination to make yourself.

When to Call the Caterer and When to Eat Out

Caterers are a hostess's best ally. Planning a shower for twenty to twenty-five people in your home is manageable, but if you are expecting more than that, weigh the cost options of hiring a caterer. They can provide china and flatware, glasses and bar equipment, and labor for setup and cleanup. More important, they can free you to be a hostess instead of the chef. Caterers will work within your budget and with your style, theme, and food tastes in mind. The caterer also has access to resources for décor, lighting, bartending, rentals, and favors.

E-QUESTION

What about guests with restricted diets?
Any caterer worth their salt will be able to accommodate guests with dietary restrictions. Most caterers will plan for one or two vegetarian meals; however, if you are aware of guests with very specific or unusual food needs, like peanut or shellfish allergies, let the caterer know in advance.

Call the Caterer

Consider a caterer when: your guest list exceeds thirty-five, you are planning a full meal, and you have limited time and access to manpower for prep work, serving, and cleaning up. When the shower is hosted by a group, the catering costs will be divided among the total number.

The best way to locate a caterer is word of mouth. Ask friends, neighbors, coworkers, and family if they have had any experience with a caterer. Get their feedback and make the call. Many restaurants also offer off-site catering, so peruse your list of favorites.

What should you look for in a caterer? First and foremost, you want a caterer with experience in the type of event you are hosting. They should have references, pictures of other projects, sample menus, and ideas. Here are some questions to help you find the perfect fit:

- ✓ Are they available on the selected date?
- ✓ Are they flexible with menu selection? Can you make substitutions, or is the menu locked in?
- ✓ Do they prepare the food themselves?
- ✓ Do they provide servers, or is there an additional cost?
- ✓ Do they offer a tasting? Is it included, or is there an additional charge?
- ✓ How do they serve the food—paper, china, glass, plastic? Will they arrange for rentals if needed?
- ✓ Do they have a liquor license?

✓ Do they provide décor for the serving tables? Can they arrange for centerpieces?

✓ Do they have a portfolio of other events like yours?

Time to Eat Out

Eating out has become a national pastime. There are restaurants that can accommodate most budgets and tastes. And restaurant showers can be a less expensive option than catering in your home. Why? Because the cost of rentals and the labor to deliver, set up, serve, and clean up is more when the staff is on the road. At a restaurant, the supplies and labor for these services are on-site.

For a standard baby shower, you will need a restaurant that has a party room or area that feels more private and can be cordoned off. Allow enough space to arrange gifts, play a short shower game, and gather to open the presents. Picking a site with a preparty area to get a drink and have a chat before the food is served is also a plus.

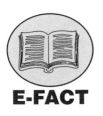

E-FACT

Try the food before signing the restaurant contract. Grab a friend or spouse and scout the site during the time frame that you plan to hold the shower. Take notes on appearance, noise, traffic flow, parking, and service. If the food for two doesn't measure up, it certainly won't get better when they prepare it for twenty-two.

It can be chaotic when the shower is winding down to its end, which makes it awkward to handle the bill. Arrange with the restaurant staff to pay the bill either in advance or in an otherwise discreet manner. Let them know when you arrive exactly who will be responsible for payment and ask about the tipping protocol—is it automatically added to the bill, or will you need to whip out your calculator? Most restaurants include the gratuity on parties with more than eight people.

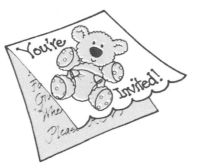

Chapter 6

Décor and Favors

MOST SHOWER HOSTESSES are chomping at the bit to dive into the fun part of party planning—decorating. Styling the baby shower can run the gamut from simply a line of yellow duckies on the dining room table to a living room completely swathed in pink tulle. The theme usually dictates the party's flair as well as the parting gift—the favors. In this chapter, you will discover some new ideas, professional decorating tips, and delightful favors that guests will love.

Basic Elements of Décor

Before you get carried away with colors and patterns, paper plates, and polka-dot linens, take the time to evaluate the areas that need to be dressed up for the party and the elements that will make your home (or away-from-home venue) look festive.

You already have determined the critical details like how many guests are coming; whether you are serving appetizers, a meal, or just dessert; and whether it will be sit-down or buffet, catered or potluck. Now you can have some fun and add the finishing touches.

Start by walking through your home or shower venue with designer eyes. Some rooms have a natural focal point, like a fireplace or bay windows. Some have dramatic architecture, while others have a cozy, comfortable look. Don't look at the flaws, look at the space. This is the canvas that you will create your shower look in and on.

Areas to Decorate

The major areas to evaluate for decorating are the outdoor entrance to the home, the inside entryway or foyer, the main party room—whether it's your living room, dining room, family room, kitchen, or patio, and the powder room.

✓ **Walkway.** Your home's walkway will welcome guests to the party held inside. It should be swept of debris and, if necessary, lit at night for safety. Luminarias—paper bags filled with sand and a candle—are inexpensive and give a warm, inviting party feel. A terracotta pot with a flowering plant or topiary or a balloon bouquet at the door also announces the festivities within. Wreaths or other door ornaments can be tied with tulle or ribbon for a simple way to say, "Come in for a party."

✓ **Inside entryway.** Once inside, guests will need to unburden themselves of presents and, perhaps, coats. Have a coat closet or rack at the ready and a designated place to put gifts. (The beautifully wrapped presents act as another layer of décor and can be moved to another room for opening if needed.) If your foyer is large enough, consider setting up a cocktail/mocktail station with a tray of drinks.

✓ **Main room, living room, or family room.** This is where the party will happen. During your walk-through you will need to consider traffic flow and conversational seating arrangements. Professional party planners often rearrange the furniture to form clusters of chairs around or in proximity to a low table (coffee table, end table, even a sturdy ottoman with a tray on top). Remove any excess clutter or delicate breakables.

✓ **Powder room.** A vase of flowers, a votive candle, interesting guest towels, an unusual soap, and a bottle of hand lotion give a bathroom a party feel.

✓ **Backyard.** Think of your backyard as another room in your home. If weather permits, bring some indoor seating outside and add homey touches like warm woven throws, colorful cushions, or interesting pillows. Don't forget to carry the theme outside by using flowers, candles, umbrellas, an area rug, and even balloons.

✓ **Focal points.** Make the most of what you already have by featuring your room's natural focal point, be it a fireplace, window, or archway. Another option is to create a new focus area—set up a seat of honor by wrapping a dining room chair in tulle, tie a balloon bouquet for added emphasis, then arrange presents nearby for easy access when it's time to unwrap them. A dining room table or food-serving table is an obvious place to spotlight and should receive special attention—a multilayered tablescape including candles, flowers, rose petals, baby items, confetti, menu cards, and the like.

Elements

Dressing up your home for the party takes many elements, all of them sensory. The use of color, lighting, and space arrangement all contribute to the creation of a party look.

✓ **Visual elements.** Once you have determined the areas that will receive your attention, look around and figure out what you have on hand that can be used as part of the décor.

✓ **Lighting.** Use light levels to create mood. A room should be well lit, but not glaring and harsh. Low lights and candles create a feeling of intimacy, which may work for a more formal dinner, an evening of cocktails, or a luncheon with girlfriends and conversation.

✓ **Space arrangement.** Traffic should flow easily. Make sure that seating is clustered and pathways for movement are clear. Allow for travel space around food-service tables, and avoid traffic bottlenecks by placing beverages and food in separate areas. Be sure to have appropriate seating for the mom-to-be and any elderly guests. Open presents in an area that will allow most people to sit or watch comfortably.

✓ **Auditory elements.** A party without music is a sad place to be; music fills in the party space. You don't need to hire a deejay for every event, but you will need a mix of tunes, a sound system, and enough songs to last for three to four hours. Music should be played loud enough to add a note of interest, but not so loud that you can't hear your own conversation.

✓ **Aromatic elements.** The power of scent is well documented. Nothing is as intoxicating as the smell of cookies baking, garlic roasting, or something browning on the grill. Equally powerful is the fragrance of flowers, candles, or perfume (however, some floral scents can be overpowering in large quantities or closed-in spaces, especially to guests with allergies).

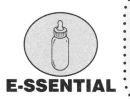

E-SSENTIAL

Teapots can be used for more than tea. Use them as interesting containers for flowers or plants. They also can be filled with potpourri and placed in a powder room or loaded with candies to reside on a coffee table.

Creating Décor that Delivers Your Theme

Now that you have inventoried your home for potential decorating treasures, you are ready to tie your shower together. Colors and baby icons that relate to your selected theme must be incorporated into the layers of party materials. When blended and mixed, these elements will lend flair and style.

Before you begin shopping for table toppers, centerpieces, and the like, take into account who is coming to your shower. Is your guest list made up of adults, grownups with young children, couples, ladies from church, girlfriends from work, or mothers and grandmothers? You don't want bone china and chintz with kids racing around the pool.

Shower Décor and the Budget

The purpose of shower décor is to enhance what already exists, not to hide every flaw in the venue space. Typically, shower décor, including paper plates, napkins, cups, centerpieces, flowers, candles, and balloons, represents about 20 percent of the total shower budget.

Most hostesses want to have the nicest possible shower they can afford. But decorating costs can add up quickly, so as with all party preparation, planning is a must. Once you have assessed your space and figured out all the decorating possibilities, you must determine what you will need to purchase or bring in to set the party mood.

Materials and Supplies

Like all parties, a baby shower does require a few special purchases to complete the event, regardless of what you choose for the theme and décor. Here are some of the basics your party will need to get dressed up for company.

- ✓ **Dishware and silverware.** If you have decided not to use paper plates and the like, you should assess your dishware. Today, an eclectic mix of good china with everyday dishes, and multiple patterns of glassware and flatware is encouraged and often gives a more interesting effect.
- ✓ **Paper goods.** If you are using paper plates and cups, they should match the décor. If in doubt, stick with basic white. Printed paper goods are usually prettier, but sacrifice looks for durability when choosing a paper plate—and avoid costly carpet and furniture cleaning from a messy spill off a droopy plate.
- ✓ **Linens.** In lieu of the standard damask tablecloths you may have in a hope chest or closet, you can use old quilts, patterned sheets,

burlap, canvas, even butcher paper as table dressing. As with all décor, layering adds interest and richness—a burlap table cloth with a lace overlay, white linen with brown wrapping paper (and tubs of crayons), will set a dramatic and creative table. Felt, designer fabrics, and tulle can all be used as runners.

✓ **Table accessories.** Candlesticks, framed menu cards, napkin rings, and place cards are perfect table accessories. Load picture frames with baby pictures of Mommy, Daddy, or siblings. A pacifier or a rattle can double as a napkin ring, or you could fill baby bottles with pink or blue jelly beans and add a shipping tag with a guest name to use as a place card.

✓ **Balloons.** Balloon bouquets are festive and pack a lot of decorating punch. Clusters up a walkway, strategically placed around the backyard, or tied to the back of each chair make the environment more festive.

✓ **Flowers.** Baby showers and flowers go well together. Consult with your florist about what is seasonally available, because out-of-season blooms can send your budget soaring. Remember to also put fresh flowers or a flowering plant in the powder room.

✓ **Baby items.** It's a baby shower, after all. Decorate with stuffed animals (then give as gifts to baby), bath or beach toys, big yellow trucks, or sweetly dressed baby dolls. Wrap baby products (e.g., wet wipes, baby shampoo, a bottle brush, sunscreen) in tulle, then cluster them together and tie with a giant bow. Voila!—a centerpiece and a gift.

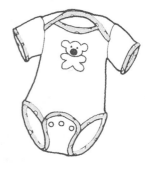

Baby Shower Color and Pattern Palettes

There are three elements of design that you can use to tie your decorating scheme into your shower's theme. Color creates a mood and unifies the party space, a mix of patterns and solids creates interest, and theme icons remind guests that this is a baby shower.

Using Color

Any color (even black) can be incorporated in the baby shower decorating theme. When using colors for party décor, avoid a smorgasbord—too many colors is visually distracting. Tie things together by using no more than three colors—a main color, one slightly lighter, and the third slightly stronger or brighter for accent. For example: Use a soft pink with white and touches of black for drama. Substitute bubble-gum pink for the pastel and chocolate brown for the black to create a trendier look.

The following table shows some traditional and trendy color palettes that you can consider in your décor. Use this table to select your color palette. Carry the color scheme through in paper goods like napkins, plates and cups, flowers, and favors.

Color Schemes

COLOR	TRADITIONAL	TRENDY
Pink	pale or baby pink with white or ivory	fuchsia or hot pink with white, pale pink, black or chocolate brown, silver, pewter
Blue	pale or sky blue with white or ivory	pale blue or turquoise blue with chocolate brown, copper, stainless steel
Red	fire engine red with primary colors—royal blue, crayon yellow, and tree green and white	Shades of red from classic red to Moroccan red, russet, Indian red, hot pink, burnt orange with black and white, stainless steel, gold, bronze, purples
Yellow	pale or butter yellow with white	marigold yellow with pewter gray, navy blue, or chocolate brown, copper
Green	soft sage or pale apple green with white or ivory	apple green or Godzilla green with chocolate brown, tangerine, Aegean blue, or lemon yellow, white or black, silver
Purple	pale lavender with white or ivory	lavender with pewter gray, aubergine, marigold, apple green, copper

Using Solids and Patterns

Patterns add interest and depth to the decorating scheme. When using patterns, the scale of the design must be considered. Large, bold graphic designs make a definitive, modern statement, but can also be overwhelming. Small floral and geometric designs work great when used with stripes and checks. As with all design, too much of a good thing is simply too much—black and white polka-dot napkins can add a perky touch, but a whole room attired in dots is dizzying. Save strong patterns for accents; use solids or subtler patterns for larger areas like tablecloths.

Using Icons

If you have chosen a theme based on a particular image or item—a baby carriage, an angel, a duck, a rattle—you may want to incorporate this into your decorating plans. You can use the icon on invitations, as part of the centerpieces, or perhaps as a featured design on the paper plates, napkins, and cups you plan to use. By using graphic software or even a color copy machine, you can incorporate cute icons into your decorating plans and put your own creative signature on the baby shower.

Décor Ideas and Projects

Part of the fun of planning a shower is showing off your creative side with some interesting baby-related décor. Many of the ideas and projects described here have the added benefit of doing double duty as both a centerpiece and a shower gift or table décor and a guest favor.

Centerpieces

The rule of thumb for a centerpiece is that if it will be used on a table where people are seated, it should be low enough to see over. Taller centerpieces can be used as a focal point on food-service tables, counters, or buffet tables.

✓ **Lollipops in pots.** Use giant lollipops stuck into terracotta pots in place of flowers as centerpieces. Pots should be large enough to balance the lollipop; usually, about 3-inch to 4-inch pots will work. Start by filling a pot with Oasis Floral Foam (dried-arrangement type), available from floral suppliers, then push a lollipop stick into the middle to create the "flower." Cover the Oasis with paper shred, bubble gum, jelly beans, lemon drops, or other individually wrapped candies. Finish arrangement by tying a ribbon around the lollipop stick.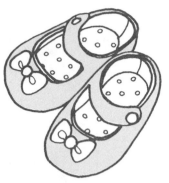

The pots can be painted in a coordinating color or be decorated with dots, stripes, checks, or other patterns. Intersperse mini terracotta pots filled with candy around the table for added punch. Variation: Use Tootsie Roll Pops or other smaller lollipops and 1½-inch to 2-inch pots to make mini pots that can serve as place-card holders and favors. Put one at each place setting.

E-FACT

The local toy store is a great resource when it comes to decorating for a baby shower. A castle for a princess shower, a jack-in-the-box or two for a Jack Jr.-to-be, giant Legos, an oversized Raggedy Ann and Andy for twins, even a doll house will be the talk of the table.

✓ **Baby bottles.** Empty baby bottles make great centerpieces and table décor. For a centerpiece, fill eight to ten mini baby bottles with pink, blue, or theme-inspired-color jelly beans, then blanket the table with them.

✓ **Pinwheels.** Pinwheels in assorted sizes are easy to make, easy to coordinate with your theme, and look festive and fun. Use our pattern to make your own with specialty paper from a scrap-booking or invitation store. When made in multiple sizes they can replace flowers.

At outdoor parties, stick them in the ground around the yard like kinetic sculptures twirling merrily in the breeze. You can also buy them online or at your local toy store. (Note: You can substitute pinwheels for the lollipops in terracotta pots described above or pop into paint cans decorated in next project. See the resources in Appendix A for purchasing information.)

✓ **Paint cans.** Available at paint supply and hardware stores, paint cans come in two sizes—quarts and gallons—and make a great container for everything from flowers to popcorn. Untouched, the silver finish has an industrial chic persona, but they can also be covered with wrapping paper or a custom label created on the computer or by hand. They are inexpensive, usually less than $2 apiece, and provide an easy way to bring your theme to the table. See Appendix C for a custom template guide for decorating the cans.

✓ **Baby-sock flowers.** Twisted and rolled from tiny baby socks, these "flowers" require minimal skills to make, but they have a big impact as well as a practical use—they can be taken apart so that the socks can be worn by baby. Rosettes can also be made from layette items, which make a fabulous bouquet for mom, centerpiece, and gift for baby. Roses can be made at-home or, for the craft-challenged, purchased online (see Appendix A).

✓ **Diaper cake or cupcakes.** The tiered tower of diapers is wrapped in ribbon and frosted with baby products like shampoo, lotion, pacifiers, bottles, and socks—and a stuffed animal or crib toy on top is a baby shower standard. Cloth or disposable diapers can be used, depending on the new parents' preference. Cakes can be created with one to five tiers, so they can become a substantial and useful centerpiece. See Appendix A to purchase one of these decorated or undecorated creations online.

Napkin Rings

When you accessorize a table, the napkin ring acts as party jewelry. Experiment with different colors, textures, and materials and go a little crazy.

- ✓ **Pipe cleaners.** Alone or in a group, these versatile little wonders can be twisted into a variety of curls and wiggles to create a festive look.
- ✓ **Ribbons.** Giant satin bows, simple grosgrain knots, or exotic wired, multilayered bows can be tied around a plain napkin for lots of impact. Raffia-wrapped linen napkins give the table an air of sophistication.
- ✓ **Pacifiers and rattles.** Slip the napkin in the ring or tie it to the napkin with ribbon or pipe cleaners. Pacifiers and rattles come in a variety of colors and can be collected and sanitized for the mommy-to-be to take home.
- ✓ **Licorice laces, candy button tape, and candy bracelets.** Tie around brightly colored cloth or paper napkins for edible, playful, and kid-inspired tableware.

Clever Favors

Sending guests home with a little present is part of the shower tradition. Although it is not necessary, it's a nice sendoff from the hostess. Favors can match the theme, and should be something that all guests, regardless of age or situation, will enjoy and appreciate. When possible, choose favors that can do double duty as both a guest takeaway and a décor item.

E-QUESTION

Should you give a favor at a couples' shower?
Everyone loves a present, but when men are involved, it is best to stay away from anything too cute or baby related. Think fun—toys like Slinkies, Rubik's Cube, Koosh balls, or water pistols are big hits. Food is also popular; candy bars, chocolate-covered pretzels, and nuts hit the mark. Sports-related items such as Frisbees, mini footballs, golf balls, as well as hand-held or desktop games will all be well received.

Food Items

Favors based on food items are possibly the most popular, versatile, and of course, yummy. Chocolate is a perennial favorite, followed by nut blends, jelly beans, and the like. A food-focused favor allows you to integrate the shower theme in the packaging, while still giving something that everyone will enjoy.

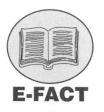

E-FACT

Many celebrity chefs now sell their products at cooking stores, department stores, and up-scale grocery stores. Ina Garten, Mario Batali, and Emeril Lagasse are just a few of the famous chefs who have developed food product lines. Designer muffin, cake, and cookie mixes, as well as secret sauces, dressings, even wines are available nationally and online.

If you choose to give food as a favor, a good way to integrate it into your shower design is to customize it. You can create personalized labels and packaging on your computer, or go online to order it done for you. A decadent jar of hot fudge sauce with a shipping-tag label stating "Share the cravings" is destined to be a hit with guests.

Consider these food-related ideas:

✓ **Candy bars.** Customize candy bars for a "sweet" shower favor or birth announcement. Easy and inexpensive, you can create your own candy bar label on the computer, download a design from the Web, or order them with customized designs either online or at candy specialty stores. See *www.everydayeventplanner.com* for candy bar art and Appendix C for instructions.

✓ **Snack packs.** Create your own signature snack mix for a unique and interesting take-home gift. Roast cashews with rosemary and place in a labeled tin, blend candied walnuts and Bing cherries for a terrific salad topper, try popcorn and gummy fish in mini-fishbowls tied with cellophane. Homemade garlic-thyme croutons in a wax-paper bag with a Caesar salad recipe, or handmade granola in a tin canister will all be high-impact, low-budget remembrances.

✓ **Specialty foods.** If sweets don't suit your shower-favor desires, consider more unusual food products. Olive oil, extra virgin or infused with Meyer lemons or herbs, is a cook's dream. Or maybe gourmet popcorn packets packaged with a list of popcorn toppers like gruyere cheese and Marcona almonds, orange zest, and semi-sweet chocolate chips. Or perhaps beverage-flavoring syrups with a recipe for an Italian soda, exotic coffees or teas, bags of pasta—they now come in unusual shapes, flavors, and colors—with for example, a pomodoro sauce recipe card. Jellies, mustards, tapenades, olives, and lemon or lime curds are available with beautiful packaging in a variety of sizes and price points.

✓ **Novelty candies.** Baby bottles filled with candy, candy lipsticks, and jewelry can all be incorporated into adorable shower favors. Margarita lollipops, lollipops shaped like dice, and classic old-fashioned swirl pops come prewrapped, so they only need a tag, ribbon, or label to say "thank you and goodbye."

Don't forget to add a customized label to your favor. They add that extra special touch. Visit *www.everydayeventplanner.com* for ideas on unique, customized favor labels.

Beauty Products

Since so many baby showers are the exclusive domain of women, beauty products are always a favor favorite. The advantage of a beauty-product present is that one or two tiny items are all you need. If you have the time, you can collect samples from the department-store makeup counters. The local mall or drug emporium carries a dazzling array of products and samples for every conceivable beauty need—from dry-skin cream and scrub to a honey-infused facial mask.

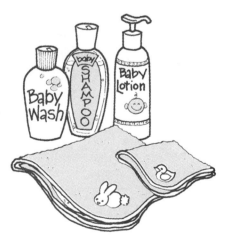

✓ **Lotions and creams.** Hand creams, eye creams, bleaching creams, smoothing creams, tanning creams, toning creams, wrinkle creams—there is a cream for everything. From fragrance-infused to fragrance-free, you will have dozens of options to choose from, including the now popular "green" products that are environmentally and socially responsible.

✓ **Makeup.** A shimmery lip gloss, a neutral-toned eye pencil, makeup-remover pads, travel-size brushes, even travel containers for makeup make great favors, and women love the idea of getting something they don't always buy for themselves.

✓ **Fingers and toes.** Manicure and pedicure products are always a good bet. Nail polishes in neutrals or fashion colors never go out of style. Emery boards—they now come in leopard, zebra, polka dots, and stripes—paired with toe separators, polish remover, or fancy cotton balls are another good favor.

✓ **Stress busters.** Anything that enhances the potential to relax is a plus. Eye masks, aroma-therapy bath products, specialty shampoos, even scented candles to put around the tub all make a splash as a favor.

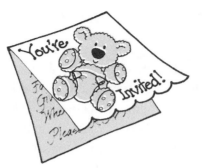

Chapter 7

Fun and Games

SHOWER GAMES DRAW either groans or grins, depending on your past experiences. If you're groaning, don't throw the idea of baby shower games out just yet. Activities, including a game or two, can be a great way to energize your party and engage your guests. Baby shower games have come in and out of vogue over the years. Many people can remember classic baby shower games like "Guess the Baby's Weight" and "Guess the Mother's Girth." When Jack and Jill showers became chic, belly measuring was mercifully abandoned in favor of Diapering Contests for the dads-to-be. Today, many showering hostesses opt for an activity instead of a shower game.

Activities Versus Games

You are pondering the finer points of whether to choose a game or a shower activity, but what is the difference? Typically, a game is short. Baby shower games usually relate specifically to babies, pregnant women, or child-care. They require minimal materials—often just paper and pen. They are designed to add an element of tradition and fun to the gathering.

A shower activity is usually more involved than a simple game. It may or may not revolve around the baby, but instead just be a relaxing and enjoyable pursuit for a group of friends. The activity can be theme-based, gender-based, or interest-based. In these cases, the shower becomes part of the activity rather that the reverse.

Popular Shower Games

Games can be loads of fun at parties! They break the ice, heat up the conversation, and get guests actively involved. There are games that relate to the party theme, and there are traditional shower games. Some games include:

- ✓ **Pin the Diaper on the Baby.** Modeled after Pin the Tail on the Donkey, this game features a supersized picture of a baby, some diaper-shaped cutouts, double-sided tape, and a blindfold. Blindfold the guests and spin them around twice. The goal is to pin the diaper on the baby's "tush."
- ✓ **Baby Trivia.** You can create your own baby-trivia cards or purchase them online. Separate your guests into two groups, each with at least ten cards. Make sure parents and nonparents are evenly dispersed! Have each side quiz the other, one question at a time. The team that has the most correct answers wins!
- ✓ **Baby Diapering Game.** For this diaper-changing relay race you need a pile of newborn diapers, four baby-sized dolls, and four packages of baby wipes. Split your group into four, or if there are only twelve women, two teams. On the mark, the first person in line must change the baby's diaper, including wiping its bottom and putting on a clean diaper. The next person in line starts the process all over again and so on, until everyone on the team has changed the baby.

Shower game prizes can be tailored to your theme (like nail polish for the spa shower) or be silly and fun. Remember, you may only need a couple. Some general ideas for prizes are: Baby Ruth candy bars, Sugar Babies or Sugar Daddies, bubblegum Band-Aids, potted herbs, bottle of wine, or lottery tickets.

✓ **Baby Bingo.** This is another game that you can create yourself or purchase. There are many themes for this game, such as Baby Gift Bingo, Baby Lingo Bingo, and Baby Bath Bingo, but the game is played the same. Using a five-by-five grid, Fill each box with one piece of information. For example: In Baby Lingo Bingo, the hostess should create a different card for each guest using about forty common baby-related words, such as binky, pacifier, bottles, bottle brush, bulb syringe, etc. Using the master list of words, write each word on a slip of paper and put it in a fishbowl. The hostess or appointed "caller" randomly pulls the words from the bowl. The first guest to get "Bingo" wins.

✓ **Mary, Mary, Quite Contrary.** Open up a nursery-rhyme book before the game and select phrases from the rhymes. Make up at least two per person for as many people as you expect (e.g., write thirty if you expect fifteen women). Give all your guests a sheet of paper and a pen. Read the rhyme aloud, for example, "The sheep's in the meadow." Each guest must write the title of the rhyme on her paper. Repeat until you've used all the rhyme snippets you collected. Have a list of answers. Whoever has the most correct is the winner. This game is also available in a ready-made version online.

✓ **The Price Is Right Game.** Buy a dozen baby items of various prices (like a package of wipes, some Desitin, a jar of baby food, a box of Zwieback toast, a pacifier, etc.). Keep a master list of the prices paid for each item. Choose three contestants at a time, and just as on the game show The Price Is Right, have them guess on five of the objects. The contestant who is closest to the exact price moves on to the next round. When all guests have played the first round, have a lightning round with each group's winning contestant to determine the grand prize winner.

✓ **Baby Pins in a Bottle.** Fill a jar with brightly colored diaper pins, jelly beans, or small candies, and have each guest write down her best estimate. The winner who is closest to the true number wins a prize!

✓ **Mother's Circumference.** This is a traditional baby shower game. Get a skein of baby yarn in pink or blue and a pair of scissors. Pass the yarn around and have each guest cut off a piece that she estimates will fit around the mother-to-be's tummy. Then, the mom-to-be has to try on each person's yarn. The one that fits wins! The best thing about this version of the game is that there is no tape measure, and no belly size revealed.

✓ **Who's Who Baby Pictures Game.** Have each guest bring her baby picture. Number and arrange all the pictures on a big corkboard or clothesline. Let each guest try to figure out who is who.

✓ **Celebrity Baby Pictures.** For variety, you might be able to find some celebrity baby pictures on the Web or in a magazine. Mingle them in with the game above, or make them into a game of their own.

✓ **Baby Picasso.** Have your guests try their hand at drawing baby-to-be without looking. Supplies are simple—a white uncoated paper plate, some markers, some lengths of ribbon, and a hole punch. Distribute plates and markers and have each guest place the paper plate atop her own head. Then let the inner artist emerge! Each guest draws a picture of baby. Give them a few minutes, and then stop to see what's been created. Pass the plates to the mommy-to-be, who chooses her favorite. You can punch two holes in the plates' edges (at the 11 o'clock and 1 o'clock positions), lace with ribbon, and have a display around the room.

Choosing an Activity or Game

Though there is no requirement to have any games or other entertainment at a shower, if you decide to play, the games or activities you choose should be carefully selected. Come up with a game plan addressing the following points:

✓ **Who is attending?** The activity you choose for a couples' cocktail party shower may not work well at a high tea shower with Grandmother and Auntie Bea. Consider the age, gender, and skill levels of your guests.

✓ **When will you play the game?** If you want to use a game to get acquainted, start as the guests arrive. Once everyone (or most everyone) is there, take a moment, preferably right after the introduction and welcome, to explain the rules of the game, the prizes, and when the winner will be announced. Other games may work best when sandwiched between the food and the presents. Games should last no more than fifteen to thirty minutes.

✓ **When will the entertainment or activity begin?** If you have scheduled spa treatments, you may need to get guests started as they arrive to accommodate everyone. Some activities, like manicures and pedicures, may take place for the duration of the shower. Others, like bowling or a speaker presentation, should be scheduled after the food is served. Allow at least thirty minutes to one hour for an activity.

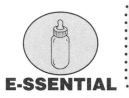

E-SSENTIAL

There is no hard and fast rule that you must have an activity or game at your shower. If you want to add an element of fun, but don't think your crowd will like a game, give a door prize for the person who came the farthest or the person who finds the hidden baby bottle first.

There are some other important factors to consider when choosing a game or activity. It should be well organized and well prepared for—have a trial run if necessary. It should create anticipation, not anxiety, and should be voluntary, not mandatory. It should have some rules, but not too many, and should be easy and fun, not a health or safety risk.

Activity 1: Setting Up Baby-Massage Lessons

The practice of baby massage is fun and beneficial for both moms and babies. You can schedule an instructor to give baby-massage lessons or use an instructional video and then practice the techniques together. It is a great activity when guests are from a play group or new mothers group, especially if babies will be invited.

To incorporate baby massage as an activity at your shower, you must consider several logistical factors. The first is environment—you will need clear, clean floor space—enough to accommodate mothers and babies. Mothers will sit on the floor with baby on a mat or blanket between their outstretched legs. If you have an instructor, she will need room to maneuver around. Given the calming nature of this activity, it is also recommended that the space be away from heavy traffic and screaming siblings. You will need equipment—a television, DVD player, boom box, iPod with speakers, or the like. Many community centers have a room available that would be a perfect venue for this activity. Finally, remember to let all your guests know what you're planning and suggest they come comfortably dressed; perhaps each one can bring her own mat or blanket.

Activity 2: Feeding Baby

Feeding baby is the number-one concern of new mommies and daddies the world over. This activity is a fun way to address this issue head on. There are several ways to approach setting up this activity. The first is to hire a professional chef to demonstrate some cooking techniques and give easy recipes for harried parents. Many cooking stores, such as Williams-Sonoma or Sur La Table have cooking facilities and offer classes. Some local cooking schools may also offer instruction. While waiting for the class, have guests prepare their own appetizers, such as sushi-style veggie rolls made with sandwich bread, or create their own open-funny-face egg salad sandwiches—a pepper smile, olive eyes, a pickle nose, and sprouts hair. Give the "Egg on Your Face" award to the most creative sandwich maker.

Another approach is to ask your guests to bring a baby- or toddler-friendly recipe and tips. Include several note cards in the invitation. After guests have arrived and had a chance to eat and mingle, have them share their ideas, then gather the recipes and tips in a decorated file box for Mommy to keep. Consider putting kid-friendly food on the shower menu—mac and cheese, peanut butter and gourmet toppings, and hot dog kebabs.

Baby Shower Arts and Crafts Activities

Arts and crafts activities are great at showers as long as they require little time and minimum skills. The best part about this type of activity is that the resulting art, usually created for the new baby, is a one-of-a-kind piece. Showers with an art activity have some space and equipment considerations, so the number of guests should be kept in mind when selecting a project to do. The space requirements will differ depending on the size of the project, but there should be work stations with adequate lighting, seating, and tabletop area. If you choose a messy project, you may want to protect furniture, clothing, or other surfaces and provide some cleaning supplies. If you will be holding your shower in a backyard or park, creating art may be the perfect touch.

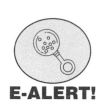

E-ALERT!

When choosing a painting activity, remember to consider ventilation and material toxicity. Certain red and blue paints have ingredients that are potentially dangerous for pregnant women. Never use oil paints or paints that require thinning with mineral spirits or turpentine. The fumes can be dangerous.

Activity 3: Painted Canvas "Baby Quilt"

This art activity yields a nursery-ready art project "brushed" by all the guests. Guests are given a small, square art canvas to paint. When finished the individual squares will be arranged and hung together to form a "quilt." You will need to purchase materials in advance at a craft- or art-supply store (see Appendix A) and do some canvas prep in the days before the party. Canvases come in a variety of sizes from 5" × 5" to 12" × 12". Be sure to buy enough canvases to form a grid. You will also need acrylic paint and a selection of brushes (you should have one brush per guest plus five to eight extras). See Appendix B for supplies and tips and *www.every dayeventplanner.com* for a painted quilt layout.

Activity 4: Teddy Bear Workshop

Who wouldn't love to make a teddy bear for the new baby? Teddy bears are easy to make, and the funny thing about them is that as they near completion, they take on their own personality. This activity is well suited to showers where the mommy-to-be has been "showered" before and has a well-stocked nursery, or for a second or third baby.

There are several ways to incorporate this activity into your baby shower. The Build-a-Bear Workshop, a national chain of teddy-bear–making shops, will host a party at any one of their stores. Bear makers can choose one of some twenty different bear styles. They then take their un-stuffed bears and make their way from the stuffing station to the finishing station, where they are fluffed and brushed. A birth certificate is issued and the newborn bear is given a dollhouse-shaped carry-home carton. And what will the teddy bear wear? You can dress your bear in everything from diamonds and leopard print to baseball shirts and sneakers. See Appendix A for Web details.

If you want to make teddy bears at home, there are kits and patterns available. To make a bear from scratch, it takes about four hours and access to a sewing machine. It is a great activity for a group of women who have sewing and craft skills. This activity can be expanded to become an entire shower theme.

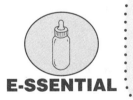

E-SSENTIAL

Giving a teddy bear a heart can be a magical moment. Purchase red puffy hearts from your local craft store. Have each guest sign one and seal it with a special wish for baby in her bear, then enclose it in the bear before sewing it up. What a wonderful gift from the heart!

Activities That Create Moments and Memories

Babies are memory makers. What better time than a shower for the guests to make a few memories, too. The following activities involve creating a gift to be cherished for years to come. These activities will be enjoyed by guests young and young at heart.

Activity 5: Scrapbook-Making Shower

Scrapbooking has taken off; there are scrapbook stores and classes, Web sites, magazines, books, and videos. The beauty of a scrapbook project is that anyone can do it. The project can be tailored to any skill level or shower theme, materials are readily available, and it can fit into most any shower budget.

Many scrapbook stores have party rooms and offer party packages. All you need to do is bring a cake and some drinks, and your shower is in full swing. You can also stage this shower at home. You will need a good size worktable—covered for protection from glue, glitter, and the like. You will need scrapbook supplies—enough for all your guests to create a page. The finished pages will be assembled in a book or binder. Your book can have a theme that matches your shower—like nursery rhymes, or the "little princess." It could also be a starter album for the new parents to document and save baby mementos and photos.

Consider these categories when creating your scrapbook pages:

✓ Home from the hospital
✓ Baby's firsts (smile, tooth, haircut, etc.)
✓ Baby's favorites (food, song, toy, pets)
✓ Look who's talking—baby's vocabulary
✓ Places we've been
✓ Baby's friends
✓ Baby's family
✓ How baby grew
✓ Gifts received

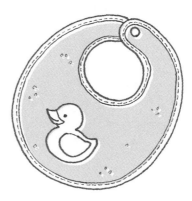

Activity 6: Parenting-Advice Book

Creating a parenting-advice book is a variation of the scrapbook activity. It can be elaborate, if you so choose; however, the advice is the only embellishment required, so it is best when kept simple. After you have served refreshments, have guests serve up their best sage parenting advice. Give each guest a sheet of paper—use a specialty paper or interesting stationery—after all, this is forever advice! Their wisdom should have a title, for example, "How I Potty-Trained Susie with M&M's," and a byline. When the guests have finished, have each one share her counsel. Be prepared to assemble the tome of wisdom in a binder or book or have it professionally bound.

Activity 7: Cards for Birthdays One to Twenty-One

This is an idea that takes twenty minutes to create and twenty-one years to deliver. Purchase birthday cards for birthdays from one through twenty-one. Give one card to each guest and have them write an age-appropriate message to the baby, child, teenager, or new adult. Collect and seal in an attractive box and present to the new parents. These cards are to be dispersed each year on the birthday. This is a lovely and loving way to gift the baby anew each year!

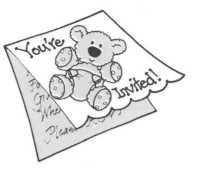

Chapter 8

Presents and Accounted For

BABY PRESENTS, like babies, come in every shape, size, and color. There are few showers that do not include the tradition of gift giving in some form. Why? Because new parents need so much that they are welcome recipients of any prettily wrapped package of buntings, booties, and burp cloths. Gifts can fill a need, fulfill a desire, create a collection, or offer unsolicited (but much appreciated) advice. From first outfit to first outing and first high chair to first year of higher education, parents have needs that friends, families, and coworkers can fill with ease.

Gift-Giving 101

Of all the shower customs passed down through the generations, opening the presents is perhaps the most anticipated. At all-women showers, the chorus of ooohs and aaahs over tiny baby booties, frilly gowns, and luxuriously soft receiving blankets is a sweet reminder of the rite of passage into motherhood.

The underpinnings that support this tradition are almost as important as the gifts themselves. As the hostess, you have to set the stage for the moment and assist the guest of honor in graciously receiving her shower of presents.

Give the Presents Presence

Guests have put thought, time, effort, and expense into their gift selection. The new mother really needs the items she will receive, and everybody enjoys seeing what's new for baby. This is a party highlight and should be scheduled accordingly. It is best to open presents either before or after the food is served, but not during. Most hostesses arrange gift opening after the food and games or activity but before the cake or dessert. Most guests assume that once the gifts are opened and a cake is served, they may leave the shower.

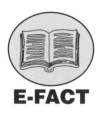

E-FACT

As each gift is unwrapped and admired, trash piles up! Have several large, handle-tie trash bags available to keep trash out of the way and gifts out of the trash. Recycle beautiful bows and ribbon by forming a "bow-kay" on a paper plate to store and use again.

Tracking

Etiquette demands a thank-you note. As the hostess, you will need to set up a system to record who gave what, so that Mommy can do her job later on. A responsible person with legible handwriting should keep track of the gift and the giver for the busily unwrapping mother-to-be so that she can delight in the gift she has received. The scribe also needs to check for gift receipts and gift certificates. Make sure there is a pad of paper and a pen for the scribe and a large envelope to put cards, receipts, gift certificates, and the gift list in; then seal it and send it home with the mom.

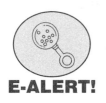

E-ALERT!

In the chaos of gift opening and packing up to go home, gift certificates, money, and the gift list can get lost in the shuffle. Have a large 10" x 13" manila envelope for cards, receipts, certificates, and such. Then seal and mark the envelope and hand it to Mom, put it in her purse, or give it to her significant other.

Finding the Newest Trends

Trend spotters and trendsetters will love looking for what's new in baby gifts. Every year, new designs emerge in the areas of fashion, style, and technology that influence the baby market. Add to that an ever-increasing understanding of health and safety issues and the changes they inspire in related products that support better baby care. There's a lot to choose from for the new arrival.

✓ **"Green" baby.** Among the most recent trends is a move to "green" baby products. Organic products are now found in many baby items, such as clothing, furniture, bedding, skin products, and cleaning products, which feature natural materials and contain no dyes or synthetics. Cloth diapers are making a comeback and with them reusable diaper covers. Green soaps, lotions, and detergents are also readily available.

✓ **Baby talk.** Babies can learn sign language. Across the country, moms and dads are learning simple hand movements that baby can understand and recreate to communicate as early as twelve months old. Teaching a baby sign language not only helps them communicate at a younger age but also helps build their receptive vocabulary. Baby Einstein, a Disney-owned company that creates videos and DVDs for babies, has recently released a new video series on baby sign language.

✓ **Dad-centric gear.** Modern dads no longer have to fear the embarrassment of showing up with a frilly diaper bag filled with impractical containers and impossible-to-button clothing. Specially designed daddy diaper bags, which look more like rugged backpacks, have places for diapers and cell phones, bottles and BlackBerries. For athletic dads (and moms) there are new kinds of equipment and dozens of accessories to accommodate baby on a bike, while jogging, or hiking. Baby hiking strollers feature wide lug wheels and a suspension system for traversing rocky terrain. Bike trailers can be attached to bikes to haul even the tiniest bundle while exercising.

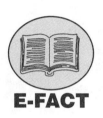

E-FACT

For the true baseball fan, a 9-inch baseball mitt can be printed with baby's name (or family name) and comes in royal blue, red, pink, or pale blue (see Appendix A). Bats, baseballs, and hats are also available for personalization. Many official sports sites now offer apparel in baby sizes, and some will add a name to a jersey as well.

✓ **Fashion for the mother-to-be.** Thirty years ago, baggy nightgowns, quilted bed jackets, and matching fuzzy slippers made a gift appearance at nearly everybody's baby shower. Maternity fashion in years past featured tents in pastels with Peter Pan collars. Mercifully, those days are history. Today, maternity wear includes body-hugging knits, belly-revealing bikinis, and low-rise maternity jeans. If you are not sure about sizes, fashion accessories, like a funky bracelet or hip earrings are the perfect third-trimester ego boost for a pregnant fashionista. Fashion magazines are great sources for trends, but search out some of the specialty publications that are devoted to pregnancy for the latest in maternity adaptations from the runways.

✓ **Fashions for baby.** High fashion has toddled into the arena of baby clothes. Designers from Ralph Lauren, Dolce & Gabbana, Versace —even Juicy Couture—have all launched lines for newborns, toddlers, and young children. Far removed from the realm of ducky-imprinted terry footie-pajamas, urban babies are showing up in AC/DC T-shirts, Led Zeppelin onesies, and Hell's Angels hoodies.

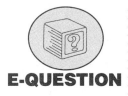

E-QUESTION

Should the hostess get a gift for the mother-to-be?
It is customary for the hostess to get the mother-to-be a gift for the shower, just like everyone else. You might want to coordinate the buying of a major gift, or you might want to give her something small but very nice just from you.

Tried-and-True Traditional Baby Gifts

Though there are certainly enough trendy, new-fangled gifts to be had, don't ignore the practical or traditional baby gifts. For people who start out weighing less than ten pounds, babies certainly require a lot of peripherals! If you don't have the time or inclination to bone up on the latest, feel free to stick with some old standards.

Clothing

Babies are born in their birthday suits, which makes gifts of clothing among the most popular, enduring, and necessary gifts for the shower. Of course, as any parent knows a growing baby will need an unbelievable quantity of outfits. Baby showers usually generate a number of outfits in infant sizes, but don't hesitate to purchase garments in bigger sizes, even up to twenty-four months. Though it's hard to imagine the little six-pound bundle wearing "gigantic" twenty-four-month-size overalls, it will happen before you know it.

A baby layette is a popular clothing gift for a shower. A baby layette consists of:

- ✓ Five to ten onesies or baby T-shirts
- ✓ Five to eight baby footed sleepers or nightgowns
- ✓ One cold-weather sleeper (if necessary)
- ✓ Five to seven pairs of socks or booties
- ✓ Three to five soft cotton pants

- ✓ One or two newborn cotton hats (babies lose body heat through their head)
- ✓ One or two Kimono-style cotton jackets (babies need to keep warm)
- ✓ Three soft receiving blankets
- ✓ Six to ten burp cloths

E-QUESTION

How many diapers will a baby use in the first year?
According to Pampers, new babies need changing up to ten times per day! As baby gets older, diapers are changed less frequently. The average American baby goes through over 3,000 in one year. When in gift-giving doubt—give diapers!

Furniture

Baby furniture is usually a large-ticket item—new cribs start at about $300. It is not customary to receive a lot of furniture at a baby shower, but it is the perfect investment if you have a group pooling funds for a gift. Obviously, you need to know if the new parents have basic nursery furniture before you rush out to purchase anything major. If you decide to make a furniture purchase, remember to check with the new parents about their style and needs, then be aware of the following:

- ✓ **Where is it manufactured?** Many countries have manufacturing and safety standards different from the United States. Make sure the materials and finishes are baby safe and nontoxic.
- ✓ **When will you receive it?** If the crib, rocker, dresser, and such are not in a local warehouse, how long will it take to get to you? What about back orders?
- ✓ **How will Mommy get this gift home?** Most retailers offer delivery service (sometimes at a nominal fee), but if you have it delivered to the shower location, can the belly-bursting mamma get that huge glider rocker in her car? You might consider presenting a framed photo of the gift to her at the shower, then arrange for delivery directly to her home some time after the shower.

Nursery Essentials

This is the standard equipment found in the modern nursery:

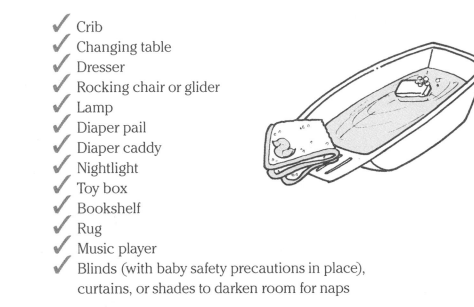

- ✓ Crib
- ✓ Changing table
- ✓ Dresser
- ✓ Rocking chair or glider
- ✓ Lamp
- ✓ Diaper pail
- ✓ Diaper caddy
- ✓ Nightlight
- ✓ Toy box
- ✓ Bookshelf
- ✓ Rug
- ✓ Music player
- ✓ Blinds (with baby safety precautions in place), curtains, or shades to darken room for naps

Toys for Tiny Tots

It will seem like a matter of minutes before tiny baby is ready to play. Infant toys, like rattles and cuddly soft dolls, will give way to play mats that will entertain baby and encourage leg and arm movement. When baby is sitting up, the play saucer will delight him and parents alike. Johnny Jump Ups, which suspend a sling seat from a doorway, can entertain even the most energetic of babies. Many toys offer the added feature of music, which babies love—look for crib toys that play a lullaby and car-seat toys that sound like a brass band. And don't forget educational toys for baby—even the tiniest ones can learn while listening to music, watching a video, or manipulating specially designed shapes that help develop coordination and motor skills.

Gift Giving with a Theme

If you want your gift giving to pack a little more punch, theme it! A gift theme doesn't have to match the shower theme, although it can. If you can't find the gift you are looking for, theme shopping allows you to create a unique gift based on a concept. Here are some idea seedlings for you to grow into a gift-giving theme:

- ✓ **A Day at the Beach.** Fill a beach bag with everything "beach," including sunscreen (SPF 50, please!), a hat, a hooded towel, stay-put sunglasses, baby cabaña, beach toys, and a sunny romper to wear home.
- ✓ **Feeding Frenzy.** Any gift that makes feeding time easier will be welcomed by new parents. Start the baby food preparation system and add a package of disposable bibs, snack containers, a no-squeeze juice box holder, a pack-and-go placemat, organic baby food, a spoon or Zoom-spoon, and the story of *Phillip the Finicky Eater.*
- ✓ **Squeaky Clean.** A baby bathtub is the jumping-off point as well as the perfect container for a bath-themed gift. Add baby bath gel and lotion, a super-soft hooded bathrobe, terry wash cloths, and a retro rubber ducky.
- ✓ **All Dolled Up.** A head-to-toe ensemble (or two) for a dressy occasion.
- ✓ **Pajamarama.** A collection of pajamas for every season and size in the first year.
- ✓ **Calendar Baby.** An outfit a month for twelve months in progressively larger sizes (this is a great gift to go in on with a group).
- ✓ **Bs in a Bonnet.** Fill a basket with bonnets, bibs, booties, and burp cloths.
- ✓ **Under Wraps.** Swaddling blankets in a variety of colors.
- ✓ **Accessories for the Nursery.** Bumper pads, sheets, coat hangers, fanciful drawer pulls and knobs, and wall art.
- ✓ **Accessories for Travel.** A car seat, diaper bag, travel suitcase, Pack 'n Play, stroller.
- ✓ **Education and Educational.** College fund, bonds, classes in music, art, parenting, movement.

Personalized Gifts

A baby gift that's been personalized with the family's name or baby name quite often becomes a lifetime keepsake. Many malls have vendors who can stamp or machine engrave a name on a gift item while you wait. Custom hand engraving may take several weeks; make sure you see samples of the hand engraving before you leave a treasured heirloom to be marked.

✓ **Born with a Silver Spoon.** Sterling-silver cups, teething rings, rattles, and spoons have long been considered the ultimate baby gift. Many items have a place for engraved names or initials.

✓ **And Now a Word from Our President.** You can send a request to the White House for a personal note of congratulations on the birth of a baby. Allow time for this gift to be received. The service is free, but the impact is worth any Benjamin, Washington, or Jackson. See Appendix A for address information.

✓ **Name That Star.** There are thousands of stars in the galaxy just waiting to be named. Send to the International Star Registry and have a legal, certified, scientific, and totally valid star named after baby.

✓ **It's All in the Purse.** If baby is already here, create a purse for mom that she'll cherish forever. Z Becky Brown can incorporate your photos into a one-of-a-kind bag that will never go out of style.

✓ **Pacifiers.** Have baby's name printed right on her pacifier at *www .itsmybinky.com.*

✓ **Blankets.** Photos and artwork can be printed on blankets at *www .blanketworx.com.*

✓ **Lamps.** With just a picture and a few weeks time, Lamps Plus can turn out a custom lamp for baby's nursery.

✓ **Art Imitates Life.** Using new computer technology, human DNA can be interpreted and printed to create art pieces. DNA 11 will take baby's DNA or tiny fingerprint and turn it into a stunning graphic design.

The Gift Registry

The baby gift registry has grown up over the last ten years. Today, almost every baby supplier and retailer has a gift registry, many of which can be accessed online as well as in the store. The advantage of the gift registry is that a mother-to-be can create a wish list of items she needs and wants. It can be a help to shoppers unfamiliar with current baby needs. Another advantage is that it can save guests hours of traipsing from mall to mall, since many retailers offer online ordering, wrapping, and delivery service. If your guest of honor has registered at a baby retailer, get the particulars (name she's registered under, the retailer, etc.). When guests call to respond, you can pass the information along if they ask.

Remember, there is no requirement to register for gifts. It is simply a way for guests to have access to some basic information about your tastes, needs, and desires. There is also no requirement for guests to purchase only from the registry. Sometimes the best presents are those from a thoughtful guest who shares something she found useful as a new parent or knew you would like it before you knew it yourself.

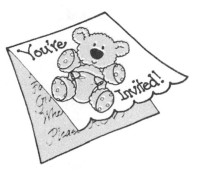

Chapter 9

Celebrity-Style Baby Showers

THOUGH ALL BABIES ARE STARS in the eyes of their parents, when Hollywood stars have babies, it seems like everyone pays attention. From conception to birth to first birthday parties, people are fascinated by the mystique of the celebrity's cravings, maternity fashions, and shower celebrations. Celebrities can afford the lifestyle that most people just dream of. Alas, if a $2,400 bassinette is not in your hostess budget, you need not despair—you can use this chapter to create celebrity-style showers that look the part but won't require sacrificing a college education.

9

Headline-Making Details

What gives a shower celebrity-style status? A fabulous location, customized details, over-the-top décor, and trendy food prep. If you're not a celebrity, but want to throw a shower like one, here are some key design elements to keep in mind as you choose the details.

✓ **3-D invitations:** Celebrities have put a new spin on 3-D for their invitations. They are dazzling, delicious, or done by hand. A flat paper invitation won't cut it on the celebrity circuit. Maple blocks, imprinted with the invitation details and artwork on all six sides are showing up around Tinseltown. Custom boxes filled with edibles—from candy necklaces to Godiva chocolates to Cracker Jack retro toys—announce the shower date and time in style.

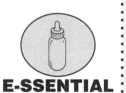

E-SSENTIAL

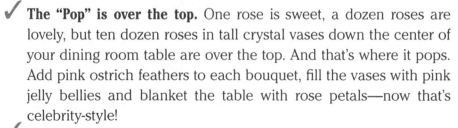

The latest Hollywood hot trends include the current hot invitation, the Egba Party Block. This invitation, a custom design by Egba Originals, can include art work, photos, and information mounted on a 2½ x 2½ inch maple cube. In the gift-giving arena, the Penelope Peapod doll comes in a bassinette/basket carry bag. See Appendix A for more information.

✓ **The "Pop" is over the top.** One rose is sweet, a dozen roses are lovely, but ten dozen roses in tall crystal vases down the center of your dining room table are over the top. And that's where it pops. Add pink ostrich feathers to each bouquet, fill the vases with pink jelly bellies and blanket the table with rose petals—now that's celebrity-style!

✓ **Work in layers.** The more layers there are, the more lavish it looks. When setting the table, don't stop at one tablecloth, use two. Then add a layer of sheer tulle. Use a square plate as a charger to set off your grandmother's antique china. Then put a menu card and a well-dressed truffle at each place—Voilà! You have created layer upon luxurious layer of style.

✓ **Expecting the unexpected.** Top designers know that to create interest, you must add a component that is unexpected. That's why leopard print and roses look so great together. Work with contrasting colors, materials, and textures to add a layer of interest.

| THEME IDEA 1 | *Under Construction* |

If a bouncing baby boy is scheduled to arrive, it's time to start building a baby shower! Use the theme Under Construction to welcome the newest member of the construction team. This theme incorporates boyish interests and fun into a party that guests will be talking about for years.

This is a great shower theme to include Dad in, so plan it for couples or family. A backyard setting will be the perfect site. Set up zones—grilling, eating, building, and gift opening—to keep the party lively. A clean wheelbarrow filled with ice is the perfect beverage bar. Load it with an assortment of beer, soft drinks, bottled water, and fruit juices. Tie a bottle opener on the handle with caution tape.

Menu Ideas and Options

A Build-a-Burger Barbeque is an easy fit for this party, and it can be tailored to any dietary preference, from beef lovers to vegetarians. Offer lots of burger-building materials or make one or two special toppers, like caramelized onions or spicy homemade mustard, to make the burgers really sizzle. Many chefs doctor up the ground meat with cheese, seasonings, rubs, even butter, but purists are happy to start with a great-quality ground steak and add their own signature touches.

Build-a-Burger Bar Materials List:

✓ **The patties.** Ground sirloin, vegetarian, turkey, salmon, ground veal, or pork

✓ **The add-ins.** Mix and match these ingredients in the ground-meat mix, for example salmon patties with dill or turkey burgers with sage or ground lamb with mint. Other add-ins are fresh basil, cilantro, parsley, spice blends, seasoned salts, sun-dried tomatoes, grated cheeses, onions, scallions, or chopped peppers.

✓ **The bread.** Classic white, wheat, or seeded hamburger buns, Kaiser or French rolls, pitas, specialty breads like rye, pumpernickel, or olive.

✓ **The cheeses.** White Cheddar, fontina, peppered Jack, Brie, Gouda, Gorgonzola. Gruyere, goat cheese, or American.

✓ **The fixin's.** Lettuce, heirloom tomatoes, avocado, purple onion, caramelized onions, jalapeño peppers, pickles, pico de gallo, guacamole, sautéed mushrooms, zucchini wheels, shaved carrots, or bacon strips.

✓ **The condiments.** Flavored mayonnaises, steak sauce, tapenades, pesto, chutneys, barbeque sauce, mustards, and of course, ketchup

✓ **The dips.** For the industrious, you can add these sauces to the bar—marinara sauce, au jus dipping sauce, ranch dressing, horseradish, and béarnaise sauce

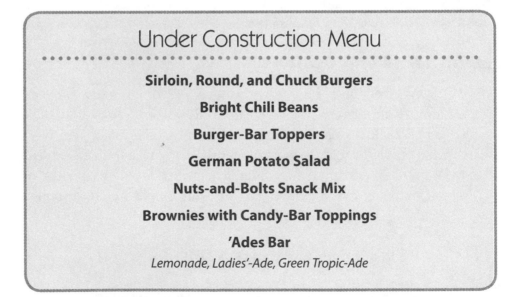

Under Construction Menu

Sirloin, Round, and Chuck Burgers

Bright Chili Beans

Burger-Bar Toppers

German Potato Salad

Nuts-and-Bolts Snack Mix

Brownies with Candy-Bar Toppings

'Ades Bar
Lemonade, Ladies'-Ade, Green Tropic-Ade

Polish off burgers by assembling a brownie—warm from the oven, topped with a selection of chopped candy bars and served with ice cream or whipped cream. Now you're done!

Color Palette and Decor

The basic color palette is blue, bright yellow (think caution tape and Tonka trucks), and metallic gray. Add touches of primary colors for interest. Hard hats, construction tools, blueprints, building materials, and big yellow Tonka trucks are the basic elements of this shower. A trip to the garage, the hardware store, and the toy store will provide all the decorative elements you will need. Cover your table with denim or burlap and add a brown paper runner. Pipe fittings provide visual interest and look great in flower arrangements set in galvanized pails. Caution tape makes great bows for the flowers. Use toolboxes to hold snacks and food such as potato chips. Shovels (new, please) become a tray for grilled hamburgers and fixings. Electrical boxes can be filled with "nuts-and-bolts' snack mix. Mailboxes, sinks, and hammers are all fair game for use at this party. Wrap flatware in napkins and use pipe-fitting clamps as napkin rings. Arrange them in a tool belt or display them in the bed of a Tonka truck.

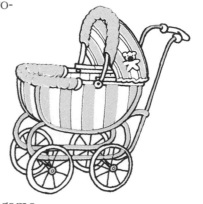

Invitation Ideas and Script

This invitation should be a blueprint featuring a baby carriage and your custom touches. The secret to the blueprint effect is to have them printed by a blueprint company. For a nice touch you can mail these invitations in tubes, which are available online or at the post office.

Baby Boy Miflin
is
"Under Construction"
And we're grillin' and chillin' to celebrate!
Join us on July 13th at 4:00
at the Rasul Construction site
14580 Riverdale Road
R.S.V.P. by July 2nd with your T-shirt size
Hard Hats Optional

The Perfect Game or Activity

Get everyone in the "zone" with this multipurpose activity. Construct your own Tinkertoy centerpiece. Have canisters of Tinkertoys available— enough to create several small projects—and ask guests to build table centerpieces. Set a fifteen-minute time limit and let the building begin. You can give awards for the biggest project, best use of color, craziest arrangement, and so on.

Gifts That Work with This Theme

In addition to the adorable baby items that every baby boy needs, there are some terrific new ideas now available. The Daddy's Diaper Dootie Tool Belt looks like a construction worker's tool belt; however, instead of holding hammers, nails, and screwdrivers, it holds a diaper, wipes, rubber gloves, goggles, and rash ointment. It is practical with a touch of whimsy.

The construction bookends from Nova Lighting are adorable as well as practical. They are a bright addition to the busy builder's nursery. Available online, they feature a bulldozer and a dump truck in primary colors and graphic shapes.

Another great gift idea is a customized tool bench. Available on the Web and at higher-end toy stores, the bench provides lots of ways to entertain the budding builder.

Favors

Send guests home with their own custom T-shirt. The design on *www.everydayeventplanner.com* can be transferred to a T-shirt, or you can create your own design.

You Will Need:

✓ All-cotton T-shirt in any color, one per guest
✓ Dark transfer T-shirt paper, one sheet for every two T-shirts (two transfer imprints per sheet)
✓ Steam iron, hard protected ironing surface
✓ Computer and laser or inkjet printer

Here's how to do it:

1. Scan design into your computer. Save as a JPEG file.
2. Print out on dark transfer T-shirt paper on your inkjet or laser jet printer.
3. Cut out design and apply per directions for transfer-paper package.

THEME IDEA 2 — *The Princess Wears Prada*

Gather the girls for a hot-pink celebration of the new arrival in celebrity style. Indulge the little girl in all your guests with a shower theme geared to big girls, too! The Princess Wears Prada is a fun, contemporary tribute to the wiles of womanhood with a touch of shopping. This theme will flip your imagination head-over-heels (Manolos, of course!) with charm and sophistication.

Choosing a location is easy! Do what the celebrities do—rent out a boutique or salon! Since the mom-to-be won't be wearing maternity clothes for long, but may not be ready for prepregnancy wear, consider hair or makeup salons, or fashion accessory boutiques—from jewelry to handbags.

One idea that's gained popularity around the nation is the purse party. These gatherings can be set up in your home or at an alternate location and combine two purposes; celebrating the impending motherhood and shopping. The premise is simple—a purse vendor sets up fashionable handbags, which are for sale, and your gathered friends are the customers. Wine, cheese, and Mocktail Cosmopolitans put shoppers in the mood. It's lively, not to mention full of great gift-giving potential—a purse-a-month for the mom-to-be.

A variation on this theme is Pucker and Pout Till Baby Is Out. For the mommy who loves makeup, this one will keep her in lipstick! Who wouldn't love some instruction for this year's smoky eyes, crimson lips, and shimmery nail? Hire a makeup artist (through the yellow pages or from your local upscale department store) to come and demonstrate to guests what's hot, what's not, and how to paint the perfect pucker.

Regardless of whether you choose to purse or pucker, invite your guests to wear something pink. It's a great way to unify the group, and it will look great in the photos.

Menu Ideas and Options

Treat your guests to sips and samples of tasty perfection served entirely in barwear. Soup shots in three refreshing flavors whet the appetite without smudging their lipstick. A fragrant garden pea and couscous salad with roasted chicken is served in a margarita glass. Demitasse cups take a shot at dessert in the form of a coffee almond float served with chocolate shortbread. Champagne may be the drink of choice for celebrities, but mom-to-be will be in the pink with Rose-Petal Lemonade served in champagne flutes.

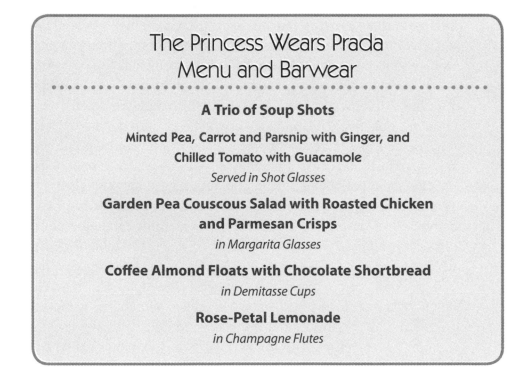

The Princess Wears Prada Menu and Barwear

A Trio of Soup Shots

Minted Pea, Carrot and Parsnip with Ginger, and
Chilled Tomato with Guacamole
Served in Shot Glasses

**Garden Pea Couscous Salad with Roasted Chicken
and Parmesan Crisps**
in Margarita Glasses

Coffee Almond Floats with Chocolate Shortbread
in Demitasse Cups

Rose-Petal Lemonade
in Champagne Flutes

Color Palette and Decor

Pink is the obvious color choice for this party, although any fashion-forward color trends can be mixed in or substituted and will create the desired designer effect. Chocolate is the new black, as they say, and it is gorgeous in combination with pink, turquoise, or pale blue. Hot lemon and lime are being paired with pink for spring. Polka dots have made a comeback and are abundantly evident on party goods as well as in fashion.

Pretty in pink and decked out is the decorating idea for this theme. Before the blessed event, collect shopping bags emblazoned with designer names or trendy boutique stores and enlist fashionista friends to do the same. Then use the bags as table décor—hide a vase chock full of pink peonies or fill a bag with a swath of tulle and tissue in two colors: For example, a small black DKNY bag (typically black and white) stuffed with hot pink tulle and pink polka-dot tissue. Think window dressing—a stack of designer shoeboxes, slightly askew and surrounded by shopping bags in varying heights. Intersperse multilevel pedestal cake plates with hors d'oeuvres. Glass-slipper vases and containers can be found online. Order several and fill with pink jelly beans or M&M's, then use as centerpieces, place cards, or favors. A variation on this idea is to decorate using baby shoes; which can also be used as part of the gifts to mommy.

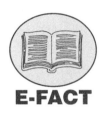

E-FACT

The perfect pout starts with red lips, that timeless fashion statement. Although skin and hair coloring are the determining factors when selecting the perfect red, these three brands are among the top sellers, year in and out: Chanel's Infrarouge in Scarlet or Rouge Noir, Dior's Diorific in Roulette Red or Dolce Vita Red, and YSL's Rouge Pur #48 or #24.

Invitation Ideas and Script

Local craft stores carry a range of shoe-shaped items that will work for this invitation. In addition, ready-to-use die-cut invitations can be found in a variety of shoe shapes and themes and are available at card and party stores as well as at online outlets.

> Our friend Missy Houghton is having a child
> So wear something pink and prepare to go wild!
> The Princess Wears Prada
> A Celebration to Welcome a New Style Star
> Tuesday, January 30th at 2 o'clock on the Loggia

The Perfect Game or Activity

Fashionistas and Prada wearers don't "do" traditional party games. Encourage some silly, but enlightening, conversation with Girlfriend Table Topic Cards, available in stationery stores and online. Dozens of questions like, "If you had to gain ten pounds what would you eat to gain the weight?" "What would the 'perfect' man be like?" and "What was the worst hairstyle you ever had?" will keep everybody laughing.

Gifts That Work with This Theme

Many fashion houses are designing for babies. From Ralph Lauren to Versace, you can find baby fashions like bibs, layettes, and blankets with designer labels. Diaper bags and other baby gear have also gone haute couture, with très chic handbag makers Coach, Burberry, and Gucci now offering diaper bags, baby carriers, and all-purpose messenger bags, even cashmere blankets for new moms and babies. In addition, you may want to purchase a copy of *This Little Piggy Went to Prada* by Amy Allen, a book of modern-shopper nursery rhymes, or one of the many celebrity-authored story books.

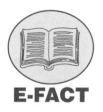

E-FACT

Many celebrities have written children's books. Among these titles are *The English Roses* by Madonna, *The Blue Ribbon Day* by Katie Couric, *Marsupial Sue* by John Lithgow, *Today I Feel Silly* by Jamie Lee Curtis, and *I Already Know I Love You* by Billy Crystal.

Favors

Give your guests a practical gift they will use every day—a lipstick mirror and mints. Little I makes a hot-pink tin filled with breath-freshening mints and a mirror for reapplying the all-important lipstick. For the shoe-crazed, pick out a collectible shoe tchotchke that matches her personality. There are so many to choose from that whether she's a boot-wearing cowgirl or a stiletto-heeled supermodel, you'll know when the shoe fits.

Roll Out the Red Carpet: A Celebrity-Style Couples Shower

The red carpet is the epitome of Hollywood glitz, glamour, and style. And no celebrity baby shower trio would be complete without a salute to this iconic tradition. Roll Out the Red Carpet for Baby: A Star-Studded Evening for Couples is the theme that pulls out all the stops for the shower in which cost is not an obstacle.

From the flash of paparazzi cameras that should announce the arrival of each guest to the Swarovski crystal-encrusted pacifier on the gift registry, this is a shower worthy of a magazine spread. Don't be blinded by the "bling." A star-studded soiree of this caliber is really a matter of attention to a few key details and the willingness to indulge your fantasies.

Menu Ideas and Options

Mom isn't the only one who will feel like a star. Score an all-star hit with this award-worthy menu. You can serve this meal buffet-style or ask guests to choose one of the three entrees when they R.S.V.P. and have the dinner plated and served more formally.

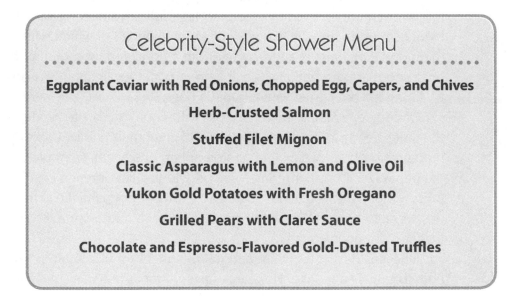

Celebrity-Style Shower Menu

Eggplant Caviar with Red Onions, Chopped Egg, Capers, and Chives

Herb-Crusted Salmon

Stuffed Filet Mignon

Classic Asparagus with Lemon and Olive Oil

Yukon Gold Potatoes with Fresh Oregano

Grilled Pears with Claret Sauce

Chocolate and Espresso-Flavored Gold-Dusted Truffles

Color Palette and Decor

Obviously, the color scheme for this shower includes red, but consists primarily of black, white, and gold. Keep the red to a minimum to allow the "red carpet" to take a prominent role at the event. White linens, white flowers, black china, gold flatware, and gold candles complete the table décor palette.

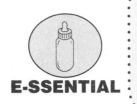

E-SSENTIAL

Personal champagne buckets are a detail that really makes the champagne pop. Purchase small bowls, approximately 3 inches deep made of glass, crystal, or silver, to use as mini-champagne buckets. Fill them with ice, add the mini champagne splits and have them passed or arranged on trays at the entrance of the party to welcome the guests.

Staging this party is the first step to creating a world usually reserved for the rich and famous. You will need a place to make an entrance—a long driveway, an extended curbside pull-up, or a grand stairway. A party like this will require an evening setting to take full advantage of searchlights, twinkle-lit trees, and the soft glow of candlelight, all of which will help set the mood. You can get a red runner from a floral supply company, theatre prop shop, or party rental store. If extreme outdoor lighting isn't possible, try lining the red carpet with luminaria bags.

Of course, walking the red carpet will require guests to be dressed to the nines, ready to meet other celebs and greet their public. Capture these moments on film by having a photographer, or several, snap pictures like the paparazzi. Consider hiring a celebrity look-alike or rent a costume and press a friend into star action to add an extra layer of panache to the festivities. Mom-to-be's arrival (limousine, anyone?) should be timed so that she makes a dramatic entrance.

Once inside, the festivities and star treatment should continue—passed hors d'oeuvres and Piper-Heidsieck mini champagne splits (packaged in a bright red bottle), served with a straw will greet each guest. Have a special bottle of sparkling water and a curly straw ready for the star mommy, who may not be drinking champagne.

In classic cocktail-party form, lights should be dim, tables draped, seating offered at varying heights, candles everywhere, and lots of up-tempo music wafting through the party space. If space allows, consider a live band with a singer to get people up on their feet and dancing. Keep the photographer busy all night taking pictures of the mom-to-be and her circle of friends. Let the gift opening begin with a drum roll from the band, and send guests home with another tradition borrowed from the Oscars—the gift basket.

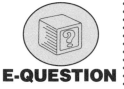

E-QUESTION

Are flakes of gold safe to eat?
Gold and silver have been used by top chefs for centuries as a way to garnish the most elegant of culinary delights. Gold has no nutritional value. It also has no fats or carbohydrates, and it passes through the body without incident. Although silver is also without nutritional value, there are occasional reports of some stomach reactions to this garnish. Go for the gold and garnish with confidence!

Invitation Ideas and Script

What is more dramatic than getting a film canister that contains your invitation to the party of the year! (See Appendix A for details)

It's the occasion we have all been waiting to celebrate!
Join us as we
Roll Out the Red Carpet
To welcome Baby Greaves
There will be Dinner, Dancing, Lights, Action, and Pictures
So get dressed to the nines!
Saturday, October 22 at 8 o'clock in the evening
Cocktail attire and maternity wear welcomed

The Perfect Games or Activity

Have your own version of *Dancing with the Stars*. A live band or deejay will help keep your party moving, but a good mix tape can also set the mood. Choose a mix of musical styles and eras from swing to contemporary, but keep in mind the sophisticated tone you will be setting.

Gifts That Work with This Theme

Considering the star magnitude of this shower, assume that the parents-to-be will want to share their progeny with the public—give them gifts that can make this dream come true. A group gift of a camcorder, a still camera, or a photo printer will be much appreciated and well used. Camera phones or digital picture frames are also great gifts. If the parents are camera challenged, consider giving the gift of photography. Give them a session with a professional photographer. You could also offer a Hollywood-style photo album from Gousman's Bookbinding in Los Angeles, which offers binding services to help compile the many new baby photos into albums.

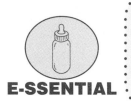

E-SSENTIAL

When putting together a musical play list, consider Tony Bennett, Elton John, Burt Bacharach, Cole Porter, and contemporary soft-rock artists such as Nora Jones, and Liz Phair. Starbucks now offers mix tapes of top artists, and you might find one that fits your shower crowd to a tee.

In the "bling" department, try a little something from Paci Posh, where they can cover everything from baby pacifiers to diaper-wipe containers with as much bling as any baby could need.

Favors

After an evening of star power, guests will appreciate the party's parting gift—a basket worthy of star status. Include a memento of the evening—a picture of each guest with the guest of honor in a picture frame. Chocolate is always appreciated: Guests will love mini chocolate champagne bottles. Custom-labeled wine announcing the impending expansion of the guests of honor would be a delicious and indulgent pleasure. Other basket additions could include Serendipity's Frozen Hot Chocolate, a foot scrub for tired dancing feet, or a soothing eye pack for beauty sleep.

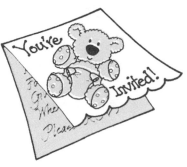

Chapter 10

Girlfriends Go Wild Shower

THESE SHOWER IDEAS may remind you of the days before babies, when the focus was primping for the prom, calling boys and hanging up, and laughing or crying over a bad haircut. Celebrate the silliness of girl talk, new hairdos (and don'ts), and the latest nail colors as you prepare to welcome the next generation.

Who Can Use This Theme

This shower concept is designed for a smaller, more intimate group of close girlfriends—whether it's the ones who had high school slumber parties; were sorority sisters and bridesmaids at each others' weddings; or met in a "work pod," exercise class, or toddler playgroup. Regardless of when and how they came together, these are the women who will move through the baby experience with the mom-to-be. So get on the phone, send an e-mail, and start planning the mother of all girlfriend-inspired baby showers.

Setting Up at Home

Having an opportunity to get together for uninterrupted gossip and giggles makes the home shower a natural choice. All three of the theme ideas presented in this chapter will work at any time of year and any time of day. The Everything Night-Night Shower could be staged as a slumber party or a morning coffee; the Playing Footsie theme can be modified for at-home set up on a Saturday afternoon or a weekday morning. The Cute as a Button shower, planned in a more traditional style, can be as simple as cake and coffee, or be converted into a luncheon on your back porch.

The key to planning for this group is to keep it small (about a dozen), get everyone involved (after all, it's friends), and keep the planning chaos to a minimum.

Setting Up Away from Home

These shower themes work great at home, but they can also be adapted for other venues. If the friends are spa girls, plan the shower at your favorite salon or resort for a day (or weekend) of celebration and rejuvenation. Friends coming in from out of town? Have a sleepover at a hotel—and go down to breakfast in pajamas and robes. Remember to allow the pregnant guest of honor to have a comfortable place to lay her head and a reasonable amount of shut-eye, since sleep deprivation will definitely be in her future!

Invitation Ideas

This invitation can be used for all the themes in this chapter. Embellish this invite with baby buttons, a tiny bow, or a dot or two of glitter, if that suits your style.

> Oh, Baby! It's a Girlfriends' Baby Shower for Sara!
> Sunday afternoon at 2 o'clock
> Poolside at Lynne's House
> Hosted by Maria, Sydney, Erica, Maya, and Jesse

For THEME 1: Come "Pedi" Ready, We're Playing Footsie! It's an afternoon of poolside pampering and pedicures!

For THEME 2: This baby's going to be cute-as-a-button! Help us create a one-of-a-kind wallhanging for Sara's cutie-pie. Please bring a special button that represents you to put on the art piece we make.

For THEME 3: We want to prepare Sara for the sleepless nights ahead at this Everything Night-Night Shower. Come in your pajamas and slippers, and bring your best baby-sleep advice and a night-night related gift.

THEME IDEA 1 — *Playing Footsie, Tootsie! A Pedicure Shower*

Pretty feet are always in fashion, and having a pedicure or manicure is a luxury for everyone, especially the mom-in-waiting. You can hold this shower at a local salon or spa, or you can create your own sanctuary and have it in your home. If you choose this option, make accommodations for someone to assist the mom-to-be, whose growing tummy may prevent her from reaching her rejuvenated feet. Whether you stage this shower in a spa or salon or opt to have it in your home, the goal is the same—a little pampering, a little chatting, a lot of celebrating, and, with any luck, no chipping!

Menu Ideas and Options

To keep everyone out of the kitchen and into the nail polish, etc., set up a salad bar. A dazzling array of fresh vegetables, fruits, and fixings allows everyone to create their own perfect dish.

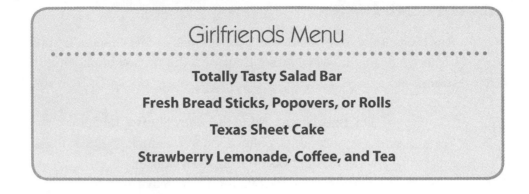

Girlfriends Menu

Totally Tasty Salad Bar

Fresh Bread Sticks, Popovers, or Rolls

Texas Sheet Cake

Strawberry Lemonade, Coffee, and Tea

Divide the salad bar ingredients up among the cohostesses with instructions to have them washed, sliced, and ready to go. Create an interesting tablescape by displaying platters and bowls at alternating heights. When assembling trays, think of the foods and colors as paint on a canvas and arrange in an artful and eye-pleasing profusion of reds (peppers, tomatoes, beets), yellows (squash, yellow peppers), greens, (broccoli, lettuces, spinach, green beans, cucumber, scallions) black (olives and beans), and white (onions, cauliflower, jicama, mushrooms) or place on a lazy Susan for easy access to all. Serve with hot bread or rolls from the bakery or grocery store. Keep the dessert simple and sweet by serving a sheet cake; it is easy to cut and serve and can be decorated with the art from the shower invitation. Bring a finished invitation to the bakery or give the bakery a computer disk with a digital image that can be printed in food coloring on specialized "icing" paper and laid directly on a frosted cake.

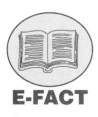

E-FACT

A standard sheet cake, available at nearly every bakery, measures 18" x 24" and serves up to seventy people. The half sheet cake measures approximately 11" x 17" and serves about thirty-five people. A quarter sheet cake is generally about 9" x 12" and can serve approximately fifteen to eighteen guests.

Color Palette and Decor

Nail-polish colors—hot pink, hot orange, and cocktail waitress red set the palette for this shower theme. Whether you are staging this in your home or at a salon, make your party pop with a profusion of girl-centric colors and patterns.

This party's decorating pop comes from flower pots planted at each "pedi" station and filled with all the "bloomin'" products you'll need for fancy feet. Using a large terracotta pot, au naturel or painted in your theme color, sprout a pair of flip-flop "leaves" and a paper magnolia with a baby button face. Also "potted" are Tootsie Roll Pops, cotton balls, polish remover, nail files, toe-separators, foot lotion, even a ladybug nail decal or two.

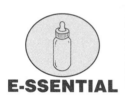

E-SSENTIAL

You can make your own paper flowers in two shakes. Use several sheets of colored tissue paper, folded into accordion pleats and tied with florist wire or pipe cleaners. See Appendix B for complete directions or search the Web for paper-flower variations.

Arrange a pot on colorful folded terry towels at each foot station. Have a bowl of roasted thyme almonds or peanut butter–filled pretzels paired with flavored water at each pedicure station for snacking.

Add pink polka-dotted lunch plates with reverse polka-dotted dessert plates and napkins or choose one of the dozens of bright patterned or floral designs now available. Add dotted confetti scattered around the food table. Don't forget to bring your iPod or boom box for plenty of toe-tapping tunes to keep the party hopping.

The Perfect Baby Shower Game or Activity

It will take between thirty minutes and one hour to complete each pedicure. If you are at a salon, the standard pedicure takes an hour and will consist of soaking the feet in a tub of warm water, softening skin and cuticles with special oils, nail shaping and trimming, scrubbing the feet with salts and salves, tissue massage, and, finally, painting the little piggies the current fashion-forward color.

The at-home version of this pedicure party may require a modification of a full salon foot treatment due, in part, to setup and cleanup requirements between procedures. For this reason, a mini pedicure is recommended for partying at home.

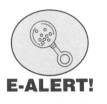

E-ALERT!

If outdoor pedi stations tickle your fancy, make sure to have SPF 30 sunscreen on hand. Red toenails are divine, but red noses are a definite no-no! Apply sunscreen to legs when you massage in lotion and don't forget faces, arms, and back of the neck.

To set up mini pedi-station flower pots you will need:

- ✓ Nail polish
- ✓ Nail polish remover
- ✓ Top coat polish
- ✓ Soothing or exfoliating foot lotion
- ✓ Foot buffer
- ✓ Toe separators
- ✓ Nail file
- ✓ Cotton balls
- ✓ Moist towelettes
- ✓ Tootsie Roll Pops

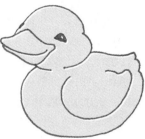

Optional: Nail decals, sun oil, and "grass" tissue paper clusters or green shred (like the stuff in Easter baskets).

To arrange the mini pedi stations in your home or backyard, simply line up chairs in two rows facing each other. Allow about 24 inches between each chair. Lay a folded terry towel on the floor in front of each chair and plant a pedi pot in the middle of the towel. Your own salon is ready to pedi. As your nails dry, swap baby stories, slip into flip flops, and "ooooh" and "aaaah" over baby gifts.

Remember to use caution when including beauty services at your next party. Keep food, beverages, and beauty products separate.

Name that Nail Polish Color, Baby!

A great game for this shower is Name that Nail Polish. For this you will need:

✓ Ten bottles of nail polish, lined up on a tray and numbered 1 through 10
✓ Paper and pen for each guest
✓ A timer or wristwatch

Ask each guest to come up with new names for the colors using the word baby or a baby reference (e.g., Shake, Rattle, and Red) in the name. Set a timer for two minutes for each color. Have guests share their name and vote on the one that best describes the color and also includes a baby reference. The guest with the greatest number of creative names wins. Winner takes all the polish home.

E-QUESTION

What color of polish looks best on each skin tone?
Light-toned skin can wear beiges, light pinks, and peaches. Choose colors in the light to medium range. Darker-toned skin looks best with deeper toned polish like reds, rusts, and berry colors, even black. French manicures look good on every skin tone.

Gifts That Work with This Theme

✓ **Baby Manicure Set.** Tender, tiny nails require special clippers, scissors, and emery boards to trim and smooth the occasional hangnail.
✓ **Mani/Pedi for Mom.** In the long weeks after baby arrives, Mommy could use some extra pampering and away time. Throw in babysitting for the perfect package.
✓ **Sock Puppets.** Designed for baby to wear on the feet, these socks have little characters on them that will entertain the toe-sucking set for at least five precious minutes.

Favors

For the at-home version of this shower, the pedi pot is the favor, since each contains a pair of flip-flops. You can embellish a pair for each guest or order them personalized with the party theme or guest name.

If you have planned a salon shower, one favor that is sure to please every guest is a take-home manicure set. One that is particularly pleasing is the Pink Polka Dot set that comes in its own purse-shaped carrying case. This chic favor will fit into most handbags and get lots of use!

| THEME IDEA 2 | *Cute as a Button Shower* |

This shower for girlfriends is modeled after the classic baby shower. It has all the elements people have come to expect at the showers they attend—lunch, a cake, some games, and gift opening. On the invitation, ask guests to bring a button that represents them to the shower, which will be incorporated into a "Counting Buttons" wall hanging created at the shower exclusively for the baby. Get creative by applying the button theme throughout the affair.

Menu Ideas and Options

This menu can be prepared and plated before the party starts. Heat the bread fifteen minutes before you serve the salad for a real aromatherapy experience.

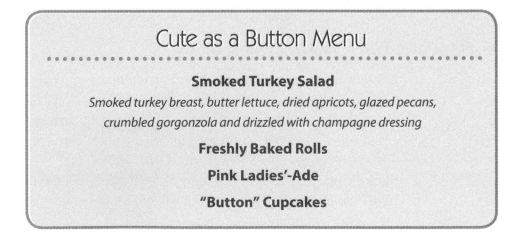

Cute as a Button Menu

Smoked Turkey Salad
*Smoked turkey breast, butter lettuce, dried apricots, glazed pecans,
crumbled gorgonzola and drizzled with champagne dressing*

Freshly Baked Rolls

Pink Ladies'-Ade

"Button" Cupcakes

Color Palette and Decor

Pastels with punch, like layette lavenders, pumped-up pale pink, and baby-powder blue, form the basis for this party palette. If you know the baby's gender, you can go with a single color, or mix the pastels if the gender is unknown. For this shower, decorations will revolve around the party's invitation design. Use the "Cute as a Button" baby icon on place cards, buttons, favor bags, and table décor. Table décor starts with a blank "canvas," a white tablecloth, runner, or placemats. Use a button stencil to create a one-of-a-kind backdrop for your tablescape. Buttons can be scattered randomly or placed in a row along the edge of the cloth or down the center of the runner. Use one or more sizes and colors to add visual interest. See *www.everydayeventplanner.com* for "Cute as a Button" art décor.

E-QUESTION

How do you make "button" cupcakes?
Start by making your favorite cupcake recipe. Color frosting to match party décor or leave white, and ice each cupcake. Form the "thread" by using black or red licorice laces to create a large X on each cupcake top. Add a dot of frosting with a plain or star tip to finish the button. Serve on a cupcake tree or "buttoned up" in neat rows on a tray.

Next, create a delightful centerpiece by applying the icon to a layette-sized T-shirt, then dress a sweet and cuddly teddy bear or two in the ensemble. Add a bow around its neck and a cluster of pastel and polka-dot balloons festooned with curly ribbons tied on a chubby paw for a table-topper and a nursery companion.

Now that the center of the table is in place, dress up each place setting. Roll napkins and flatware together and finish with a strip of old-fashioned candy "buttons," available at most candy stores.

Place a custom-wrapped candy bar at each place to use as both décor and favors and, perhaps, a mid-meal munch!

The Perfect Baby Shower Game or Activity

Any of the traditional shower games will work for this party—see Chapter 7 for a list of games, ideas, and prizes. If you want to incorporate a more specific activity, how about a craft project? The "Counting Buttons" nursery wall hanging is the perfect complement to this theme. A felt or fabric banner features ten squares approximately 6" × 6" in size. Each square contains a number from 1 to 10 and has the corresponding number of related buttons—one ball, two bunnies, three ducks, four fire trucks, and so on. Squares are marked with rickrack, ribbon, or cording. The project is made ahead of time and completed with the addition of signature buttons from each guest (as requested on the invitation) on a strip across the bottom of the wall hanging. See *www.everydayeventplanner.com* for directions on the Counting Buttons project.

Gifts That Work with This Theme

Give guests a little challenge by suggesting that the gifts begin with the letter *B*. Some examples are Boppies, binkies, bassinettes, and blankets, not to mention bottles, bedding, and baby banks.

Favors

Cute as a button, sweet as a candy bar. These yummy favors are a cinch to make, and serve double duty as table décor. Some specialty grocery stores carry a one-pound chocolate bar that's a huge treat, but even the standard size makes a delicious statement. The technique is simple—unwrap purchased bars, then rewrap in aluminum foil. Print out paper wrappers from your computer, and slip around the chocolate. A little double-stick tape and you're the candy man!

THEME IDEA 3   *Everything Night-Night Shower*

There are several ways to throw an Everything Night-Night Shower—as a retro slumber party (at home or at a hotel) or as a come-as-you-are surprise breakfast. Since the formula for sleeping baby is sometimes as elusive as the Holy Grail, why not turn the focus of celebrating to this all-important activity? Girlfriend guests will love the idea of wearing pajamas and slippers instead of skinny jeans and stilettos. If a sleepover won't work, consider breakfast-for-dinner or try the breakfast surprise version—enlist the help of the daddy to be and arrive on the doorstep to escort the mom-in-waiting to the shower site—in her pajamas. Make sure everyone else is similarly dressed—it's comfortable and a great story for the baby book!

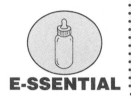

E-SSENTIAL

Every girl needs a little chocolate! Get a jolt from steamed chocolate shots instead of java. Try white hot chocolate, peppermint hot chocolate, or Mexican hot chocolate (made with chili powder) for a twist on an old favorite. Have a tray of fixin's like marshmallows, cinnamon sticks, peppermint sticks, shaved chocolate bars, and whipped cream.

Menu Ideas and Options

Breakfast can be served anytime, especially if you do a little preparation the day before and make use of your grocery store's frozen food section. Remember, you're among friends—let everyone help and leave the worries at the door. Real men may not eat quiche, but girlfriends love it. Save your sanity and hit the frozen food aisle for a bite-size version of the French favorite or try the crustless version listed here.

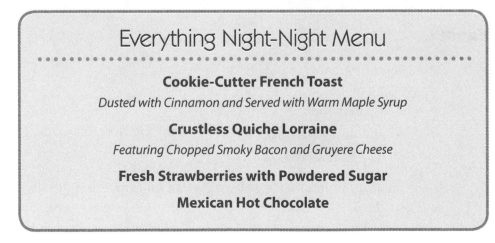

Everything Night-Night Menu

Cookie-Cutter French Toast
Dusted with Cinnamon and Served with Warm Maple Syrup

Crustless Quiche Lorraine
Featuring Chopped Smoky Bacon and Gruyere Cheese

Fresh Strawberries with Powdered Sugar

Mexican Hot Chocolate

Color Palette and Decor

This shower is more about creature comforts than décor. Instead of table décor, try individual tables in the form of TV trays. Set up each tray like a breakfast-in-bed tray with a napkin, party ready with a pacifier-shaped lollipop attached with curling ribbon. Baby roses and baby's breath in miniature bud vases and a pair of reflexology sleep socks (which is also the favor) complete the picture.

Grab gossip magazines and several seasons of *Friends* or other favorite television shows to watch while reminiscing about the days before kids. Crank calls and Ouija board optional.

The Perfect Baby Shower Game or Activity

The ancient art of reflexology is a therapeutic healing system that creates balance and well-being throughout the body. A gentle pressure is applied to specific points on the sole that tap into the body's energy. Allow guests to experience the restorative powers of reflexology with a relaxing foot self-massage guaranteed to induce a restful night's sleep. Use the reflexology slipper-sock favors to find your own pressure points.

Gifts That Work with This Theme

This is the easy part—anything that will enhance sleep for mommy or baby will work.

Favors

- ✔ Pajamas for baby
- ✔ Nursing nightgowns
- ✔ Nursery monitors
- ✔ Crib mobile
- ✔ Bedding
- ✔ Soothing music
- ✔ Night lights
- ✔ Custom painted "Do Not Disturb" door hangers

A pair of reflexology slipper socks, the kind that show a diagram of the foot's pressure points on the sole, will work for both the suggested activity and as a favor. Other ways to say thanks for coming are with little night-night treats for the guests—sleep masks, a soothing lavender neck wrap, or an aroma-therapy spray all make great favors.

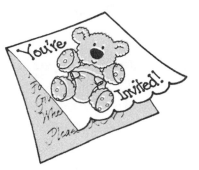

Chapter 11

Zen Tea Shower

AS THE NEW MOTHER PREPARES for the birth of her baby, friends and family can balance the impending chaos with a calming Zen Tea Shower. You will not find a scone, floral chintz, or a cup of English tea at this tea party. The style of this shower is minimalist, meditative, and serene. Steeped in tradition, the tea ceremony celebrates harmony, respect, and tranquility, which are the perfect sentiments for a baby shower. If you elect not to incorporate a formal tea ritual, your shower can still be planned and carried out in this atmosphere of calm and balance.

Who Can Use This Theme

Women enjoy the concept of a tea party in any form because at its core, the purpose is to visit and engage in conversation and the sharing of stories. This party is no exception, and as such is designed primarily for an all-women guest list. It will appeal to a wide range of ages, and with the many possibilities for participation in the tea tasting or the other activities presented here, it will reveal the wisdom of the ages. Tea bars are the hip, younger cousin to the tea rooms of your grandmother's day.

Setting Up at Home

The perfect home setting for this party starts with a clean, uncluttered environment. An indoor or outdoor area can accommodate this event. Depending on the ages of those on your guest list, and the trimester your guest of honor is in, you may consider staging the event on cushions on the floor around a low coffee table. You will also need some floor space or large table spaces to incorporate the Baby Swaddling project or Mommy and Me Yoga instruction.

Cushions and throw pillows can provide both seating and décor. Natural materials—bamboo, stones, silk and linen, and teak wood are common elements that can be incorporated into the atmosphere of this shower. If you choose to stage a traditional ceremony, but do not feel knowledgeable about its intricacies, consider hiring a "Tearista" (a barista for tea service). There are also books and Web sites that give tea ceremony instructions in great detail.

Setting Up Away from Home

Tea houses, tea shops, and tea bars are popping up all over the country, and many have party or ceremony facilities. If you can't find a specialty shop, choose a location with a meditative feel, such as a Japanese garden, a yoga studio, an art gallery, a health club, a day spa, or a dim sum house. The most important feature of the facility is that it help to establish a sense of balance and calm for the party; however, any room that fits that order can be decorated in Zen fashion.

If you choose an activity that requires floor space, such as the Mommy and Me Yoga class, take this into consideration when selecting a site. The baby-swaddling activity requires the use of the floor or a table, and the belly-casting activity will require access to water. All of these suggested activities may require the use of a DVD player to assist in the instruction, so consider power-source options or opt for a live demonstration with a teacher.

<table>
<tr><td>THEME IDEA 1</td><td>Tranquili-Tea Baby Shower</td></tr>
</table>

Satisfy your yen for Zen with this take on the baby shower. If you are staging this at home, consider using your backyard. Lotus candles and water lilies floating in bowls (or in a pool, if you have one) will add serenity to the décor. The party attitude is peaceful and joyful—a perfect environment to welcome baby!

Menu Ideas and Options

An enlightened menu that balances savory and sweet, cold and hot, spicy and mild is the food philosophy for this party. Asian-inspired foods are a good starting point for selecting a Zen tea menu, and small bites are the order of the day, so choose a variety of dishes. Dim sum consists of a variety of tiny dumplings, steamed buns with fragrant fillings, and fried rolls, all served with flavorful dipping sauces.

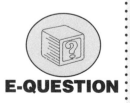

E-QUESTION

How do you brew a perfect cup of tea?
Perfect tea starts with cold, fresh water placed in a kettle and heated. Preheat the teapot by filling it with boiling water first, then pouring the water out. Add more hot water and the tea bags or tea-leaf-filled infuser to the second batch of water. For black tea, water should be brought to a full rolling boil (212°F), for green tea a cooler 185°F is needed. Pour the hot water over the leaves and allow to steep.

Setting Up a Tea Bar

Tea is for trendsetting, and it starts at the hub—the tea bar. For this shower, you can create your own version of a tea bar to educate and expose guests to the culture and delights of tea. Retail tea bars generally offer tastings from each of the tea categories—black, green, white, oolong, herbal, and rooibos, in addition to tea blends—tea brewed with fruit juice (tisanes) or spices (chai). A tea bar offers guests an opportunity to sample many kinds of tea at one sitting. There are hundreds of teas to offer your guests; however, you can keep it simple by limiting the tasting choices to six.

Zen Tea Menu

Miso Soup Shots

A Delicate and Flavorful Broth Served in Chinese Teacups

Chilled Steamed Soy Beans Tossed with Sea Salt

Spicy Shrimp Potstickers

Thin Dumplings browned and steamed with a Filling of Shrimp, Ground Pork, Bamboo Shoots, Carrots, and Chinese Mushrooms

Cilantro Chicken Dumplings

Fragrant Cilantro-Infused Chicken Wrapped in Dough

Shrimp and Green Onion Dumplings

Sweet Shrimp, Chinese Cabbage, and Green Onions

Spring Rolls

Tender Young Bean Sprouts and Pork Tenderloin Cooked in Won-ton Wrappers

Fried Bowties

Deep-Fried Wonton Wrappers, Twisted and Tossed with Powdered Sugar

Personalized Fortune Cookies and Mochi Ice Cream

You should plan on making a pot (or two) of six different teas. Tea bags or loose tea can be used, but if you plan to "read" the tea leaves, you will need loose tea. You will also need:

- ✓ **Sweeteners.** Sugar, demerara sugar (a coarse raw sugar), honey, honey straws, and sugar substitutes
- ✓ **Cream or milk.** Black, chai, and Boba teas are served with milk.
- ✓ **Teacups.** If you are planning a tea tasting, try using Chinese-style teacups like those found in restaurants.
- ✓ **Kettle.** Tea must be made with boiling water, not tepid tap water. Use either a whistling tea kettle or an electric tea kettle.
- ✓ **Optional: Black tapioca pearls.** These "beads" of tapioca have the consistency of gummy bears and are slightly larger than a pea. They sit in the bottom of the cool, milky Boba tea and have a sweet flavor. Serve this tea, which is also called "bubble" tea, with a wide straw to enjoy the pearls. (See Appendix A for pearls and straws.)

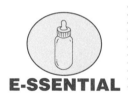

E-SSENTIAL

Tea gets its flavor from a process called steeping, which occurs when hot to boiling water is poured over the leaves and allowed to sit for a few minutes. Steeping times for teas vary: Black tea should steep for five minutes, oolong takes three to six minutes of steeping, and green tea needs two to four minutes to steep.

Invitation Ideas and Script

Simplicity is at the heart of the Zen-inspired shower invitation. Incorporate natural fibers and textures into design elements. Print the details on recycled paper, then mount on textured or linen-wrapped cardboard. Add a fiber ribbon and enlighten your guests.

Come join us for
Tranquili-tea
A peaceful and harmonious celebration
To shower Jenny
With good wishes for motherhood and baby-to-be
On the Tea Terrace at Sheri's
Saturday, June 15th at 11 o'clock in the morning
Tea Tasting, Tasseography, and Dim Sum

Color Palette and Decor

Use soft earth tones of sage green, gray, and almond, with a pop of color like apple green or plum. Natural textures and colors are the order of the day. Earth elements, such as water, fire, clay, and wood, make a strong, yet restful and meditative, statement. Bamboo, wood, polished rocks, and green plants work well together to create the right mood. Setting a table with bamboo plates (which are also eco-friendly), a long, low centerpiece of wheat grass, a bonsai tree, a waterscape fountain, and lots of green tea candles will inspire the tranquility needed for this shower. Curly, green bamboo shoots in clear vases lined with river rocks make an excellent centerpiece and can also be sent home with guests as prizes.

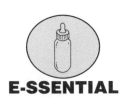

E-SSENTIAL

Looking for the right musical "vibe" for your Zen shower? Try your local metaphysical bookstore. They will carry alternative music and have a selection of artists and play lists that will set the right tone. Mega-bookstores also carry CDs in this category. You can find Zen music by searching on iTunes and other online music sources.

The Perfect Game or Activity

Don't Dawdle, Learn to Swaddle! Swaddling is a skill that's a must for new moms, so it is the perfect activity if the guest list includes other new moms or moms-to-be. When baby's crying can't be comforted by feeding, burping, or a diaper change, try swaddling. This ancient technique turns chaos into tranquility by blanketing baby in bundled comfort. Swaddling is similar to origami, and there are a number of books available on the topic. There are also organizations of "Babywearers" (see *www.babywearers.com*) who offer practical advice from nurses and other experts. To learn this technique at the shower you will need:

✓ Floor or table space with room to lay a small baby blanket flat
✓ Life-size baby dolls—one for each pair of guests (or the real thing if your shower guests are new moms themselves)

✓ A swaddling blanket for each doll
✓ A swaddling trainer or leader to walk guests through the steps and swaddling styles
✓ A swaddling book or DVD

Allow about forty-five minutes to learn and practice this technique. If the crowd relishes a challenge, finish the session with a "swaddle-off," a timed swaddling competition. Choose one swaddling wrap technique, have participating guests at the ready, and start the clock. The first guest to finish should yell, "It's a Wrap!" when they are done. To the winner goes the spoils—a bag of Tootsie Rolls in a Chinese food container.

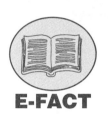

E-FACT

Tea infusers are needed when using loose tea leaves to make tea. They come in a variety of shapes and sizes and can be made of a number of materials from stainless steel to ceramic to bamboo. Look for infusers that include dip bowls or trays to make draining the tea leaves easier. They can be found in specialty stores, coffee houses, and grocery stores.

Tasseography

Another activity option is tasseography—the art of reading tea leaves. A form of fortune telling, this Eastern tradition will be a much-talked-about highlight of any tea-related party. Best of all, this activity requires little setup space and can be taken on the road if your shower is not in someone's living room. You will need:

✓ Loose-leaf tea (tea leaves that are not prebagged). Choose tea leaves that are somewhat coarse with little tea-leaf dust. Chinese teas work especially well.
✓ Tea cups with plain white interiors and wide brims
✓ Teapot
✓ Teaspoon
✓ Symbols list, one for each guest
✓ Tasseographer (amateur or professional)

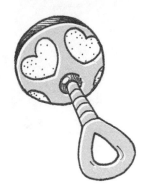

Follow these instructions for how to get ready to read tea leaves:

1. Boil a kettle (or more) of water and pour over loose tea in a teapot. Steep for two to three minutes.
2. Pour tea into cups. Do not use a strainer! Leaves will sink to floor of cup. Let tea cool to almost room temperature.
3. Have guests drink their tea, leaving some liquid and the tea leaves in the bottom of the cup.
4. Tell guests to pick up cup in their left hand, cover the top of the cup with their right hand, and swirl the cup around clockwise three times. Make sure that the liquid is swirled up the sides of the cup.
5. Have guests gently place cups down on saucer. Tea leaves will form clumps around the sides and bottom of the cup. The clumps will form patterns that will be interpreted according to the symbol chart.

There are many Web sites and books that cover tasseography in detail. Here are the highlights of tea leaf reading:

Reading the Brewed Tea:

✓ Bubbles on the surface of the tea means that money is coming your way.
✓ Floating tea leaves means visitors will be coming.

Reading the Tea-Leaf Clump Shapes:

✓ Triangles mean good karma.
✓ Squares mean proceed with caution.
✓ Circles mean success is coming.
✓ Letters usually refer to names of friends or relatives.
✓ Numbers usually refer to time—days, months, or years.
✓ Other shapes—animals, fruits, common objects such as coins—all have specific meanings in tasseography. For a complete list of Web sites, see Appendix A.

Reading the Location of the Tea-Leaf Clumps:

✓ Brim—life-change matters of importance
✓ Side of cup—significant occurrences that are not life changing
✓ Bottom of the cup—things that are subject to change

E-SSENTIAL

Many tea rooms have tasseographers available for parties as well as on a regular schedule. Ask when they are available and consider planning your party's time around this activity.

Gifts That Work with This Theme

The theme "Tranquili-tea" says it all—this shower is about comfort and calm. Gifts that are soft, warm, and cozy are the order of the day. Consider these items when you plan for a Zen shower:

✓ **Swaddling Blanket.** These blankets now come in many shapes and sizes.
✓ **Moses Basket.** Bedecked in bows or bold yet simple, the baskets are perfect for a quick nap or a longer snooze in a warm sunny spot next to mom.
✓ **Skin Products.** Many spas now offer a version of the skin products in a baby line. Look for soothing diaper-rash ointments, massage lotions, and bath soaps made from organic ingredients.
✓ **Hug-a-Bear.** A soft teddy bear is always comforting. Infants need one with sewn-on, rather than plastic, eyes and nose and no movable parts.

Favors

For tea lovers, there is no greater gift than a delicious brew. Create a take-home tea party by selecting a flavorful blend and packing it to go. This simple idea can be purchased, or you can create a handmade version. To create your own take-home tea party, you will need:

- ✓ Four to six tea bags for each guest (many tea companies now use a higher-quality mesh tea bag that looks great in the favor bag.)
- ✓ Clear cellophane gift bags
- ✓ Bag topper
- ✓ Stapler
- ✓ Computer and printer

See *www.everydayeventplanner.com* for an example of this favor.

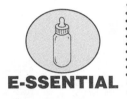

E-SSENTIAL

Tea-leaf clumps in the shape of a baby means something new is going to come to you. A duck means money is coming, a leaf means a new life is on the way, a rabbit means bravery, an ear means good news, and a cloud means wishes will come true.

THEME IDEA 2 | *Belly Bump Shower*

This variation of the Zen shower features teas of India and an interesting blend of Indian spices under the influence of British tradition. The flavors and colors of the rich Indian culture add a taste of the exotic to this version of the baby shower. The activity—painting the mom's belly with henna and giving henna tattoos to the guests, will carry out an ancient tradition and carry forward a meaningful experience for mom and guests alike.

Invitation Ideas and Script

Welcome the new little Darjeeling with an invitation that pictures a baby in a teacup.

Celebrate the Belly Bump!
Hilary's having a Baby and We're Having a Party
To Welcome Her Little Darjeeling!
Sunday, March 4th at 5 o'clock
A Traditional Indian Feast will be followed by
Henna Tattoos and Belly Decorating

Menu Ideas and Options

In Indian culture, it is believed that a perfect meal consists of foods and seasonings that produce six distinct tastes—sweet, sour, salty, spicy, bitter, and astringent. Darjeeling and Chai add flair and punctuate the tea service.

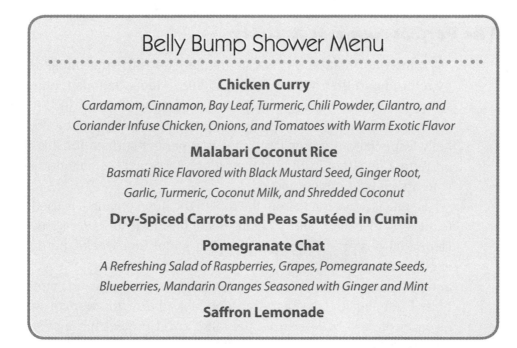

Belly Bump Shower Menu

Chicken Curry
Cardamom, Cinnamon, Bay Leaf, Turmeric, Chili Powder, Cilantro, and Coriander Infuse Chicken, Onions, and Tomatoes with Warm Exotic Flavor

Malabari Coconut Rice
Basmati Rice Flavored with Black Mustard Seed, Ginger Root, Garlic, Turmeric, Coconut Milk, and Shredded Coconut

Dry-Spiced Carrots and Peas Sautéed in Cumin

Pomegranate Chat
A Refreshing Salad of Raspberries, Grapes, Pomegranate Seeds, Blueberries, Mandarin Oranges Seasoned with Ginger and Mint

Saffron Lemonade

Color Palette

The same natural textures and colors of nature can serve as inspiration for this shower, but add a pop of color and a layer of richness to capture the robust flavor of Indian culture. Jewel-tone colors found in the bazaars and marketplaces mix with the earthy colors of nutmeg, cinnamon, cumin, tamarind, and cloves to form the palette basics. Throw in a touch of gold and silver by using bangle bracelets as napkins rings—simply drape the folded napkin through the bracelet like a towel holder to complete the look. Consider using a sari as a tablecloth and arrange wooden candlesticks in assorted heights and designs. Madagascar or night-blooming jasmine, pink or orange freesia, and sweet alyssum with the fragrance of warm honey are all excellent choices. To create a centerpiece, start with a large, clear vase and fill it with kumquats or key limes. Add a spray of russet or plum-colored orchids, add water to cover the fruit, and voilà—a centerpiece is born. Or try this fragrance-infusing trick—place approximately 2 inches of whole cloves or cinnamon stick around the base of the candle. As the candle melts and burns, it will release the aroma of fresh spices.

The Perfect Game or Activity

Bring the tradition of intricate henna tattoos to your circle of friends by returning to the roots of Eastern culture. Henna tattoos require a little setup, but they are so beautiful that your guests will be thrilled to try out this new technique. Traditionally, the hands and feet are tattooed, but the belly, especially the pregnant belly, is a perfect surface for this timeless art form. Check out local resources for professional henna tattoo artists in your area if your budget allows.

Henna is a dye made from the root of the henna plant. It is used to color textiles, to dye hair, and to paint beautiful, intricate tattoos on women. Henna tattoos are temporary—they last about four weeks, but fade after each washing. The designs are based on nature—flowers, earth elements, and animals—but some of the designs relate to religious and spiritual symbols. Hennaing is considered a good-luck charm for women who have given birth. It is believed that the tattoos will protect the mother as she recovers from the rigors of childbirth.

Henna tattoo kits are available online. They are inexpensive to order, and they come complete with directions, transfers, ink, and a pen. All you will need to provide is a willing spirit.

Gifts That Work with This Theme

As with the Tranquili-Tea shower, the Indian version is about balance and a sense of calm. Start baby out early with gifts like:

✓ **Mommy-and-Me Yoga Membership.** Yoga for babies is the newest old-fashioned way to teach movement, balance, and breathing, as well as baby massage. Classes are available around the country at yoga centers, health clubs, and even church halls. Whether you give a single class or a series of classes, this gift will help balance new responsibilities.

✓ **Baby-and-Me Yoga Clothes.** These adorable onesies and T-shirts are designed to be worn by the babies of yoga moms. See Appendix A.

✓ **Yoga Mat and Diaper Bag.** Let the new mom stretch in style with a matching yoga mat and bag (which can double as a diaper bag).

Favors

Send guests home with a taste of the party with the Chai and Chocolates Gift Bag. Handmade chai tea mix (see recipe in Chapter 19) packaged with a dark chocolate bar is delicious anytime.

THEME IDEA 3 | *Tea for Two Shower*

All babies aren't the same, and neither are all showers. Sometimes the very simplest of plans is the best and only way to proceed. The Tea for Two Shower embraces the idea of showering a mom-to-be with affection and a present or two, without the hoopla and chaos of the bigger, bolder parties. This shower theme is perfect for an officemate, an out-of-town girlfriend, or a mommy-in-waiting who has been confined to bed rest. With very little notice, and even less formal planning, this shower can spring up anywhere, at any time, for any budget, and still be something to remember.

Menu Ideas and Venue Options

For starters, select a venue—easy since the guest list is you. Choose a favorite restaurant, a local coffee house or tea room, your living room, her bedside, either kitchen—wherever it is most convenient. Décor should be at a minimum if at all—a bud vase and matching napkins, and perhaps a nice view are all that is needed.

Since the goal of the shower is to be portable, consider Chinese take-out, a Japanese bento box, or Thai pizza to go. If you are bringing the shower to mom, a bento box is a great solution to serving take-out food with style; it contains samples of several types of food, such as teriyaki chicken, steamed rice, pickled ginger, and edamame in neat compartments. You can order bento boxes and fill them yourself or have them prepared to go from your favorite local restaurant. Although Japanese in origin, you can even serve up an Italian pasta or antipasto medley in these stylish containers. Complete the meal presentation with bottled green ice tea or the Green Mint Mar-tea-ni, and serve moshi ice cream for dessert. These frozen confections are made from bite-sized servings of green tea ice cream wrapped in a sticky rice paste. They come in pale green and pink.

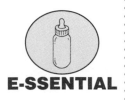

E-SSENTIAL

The Green Mint Mar-tea-ni is a teetotaler's drink, but can be made with alcohol. For two drinks, use 10 mint leaves, 4 teaspoons of simple sugar syrup, 4 lime slices, 1 teaspoon of rum flavoring, 2 cups of hot green tea, and honey to taste. In a bowl, muddle (pound gently together) mint in simple syrup with lime slices. Add the rum flavoring, then pour steaming green tea on top. Sweeten with honey to taste, then chill and serve.

The Perfect Activity and the Perfect Gift

The "bump" has become fashionable, and pregnant women everywhere are reveling in their blossoming beauty. Immortalize the bump with a belly casting. It doesn't require great skill, but there is a certain amount of disrobing that makes it less convenient in the presence of a crowd, thus making it the perfect activity for you and a girlfriend to share at home. It can also be a little messy, but most kits come with a drop cloth for easy cleanup.

Belly casting is done by placing overlapping strips of wet plaster and gauze across a mom's Vaseline-coated belly and torso. When the plaster has set, the result is an impression of the pregnant belly that will be a lasting memento of this special time. The cast can be displayed as is or painted or decorated.

Belly-casting kits are available online and in stores. They are nontoxic, safe to use on the new mom, and take only thirty minutes to make. Grab some magazines or a favorite movie to entertain yourselves while you wait for the plaster to dry. The best part is that the belly cast is also the perfect gift. What a wonderful way to celebrate motherhood, and welcome baby!

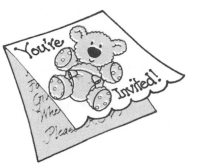

Chapter 12

A Grandparents' Shower

GONE ARE THE DAYS when the term "grandparents" referred strictly to the gray-haired couple, gently rocking the remainder of their lives away on the front porch. Yesterday's baby boomers are today's grandparents. These new grannies and gramps are far more likely to be working, traveling, finishing a college degree, or embarking on a second career. They are on the go, and grandbabies are welcome to come along for the ride. The Grandparents' Shower is a twist on the traditional shower. And while "baby" is still the lucky recipient, the focus is on the soon-to-be nana-and-papa rather than the mother-to-be.

Who Can Use This Theme

When a baby is born, so too are a set of grandparents. Fortunately, friends and coworkers can step in to bring them up to speed on bringing up a twenty-first-century grandbaby. Whether this is a first grandchild, the seventh, or seventeenth, it's a perfect time to celebrate. The idea behind this shower is simple—celebrate the impending birth (or rebirth) of the grandparents. The guest list can include women and men. The mommy- or daddy-to-be will be invited, of course, but if time or distance keeps them away, baby will still benefit from the shower of good wishes and gifts, albeit at Grandma's house. It will work at any time of year, can be held indoors or outdoors, and, since it is for the grandparents, it does not need to be in geographic proximity to the grandbaby.

Anyone can throw a grandparents shower. With Grandma out in the workforce, her coworkers may want to help her celebrate her new impending status change, but they don't know her daughter or daughter-in-law. This is the perfect opportunity to honor her and have some fun. What better way for adult children to say thank you to their parents than by gathering together and "showering" Mom and Dad with a party. Friends can shower friends—especially if you have been through the various life stages together, from newlyweds to new parents, from preschool to graduate school, and from birthday parties to weddings. Now, your circle of friends shares the experience of watching your children become parents—a party opportunity no one would want to miss.

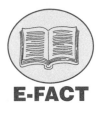

E-FACT

Did you know that the average age of first-time grandparents is forty-eight? About one-third of American adults are grandparents. Most people will be grandparents for over forty years! These grandparents are also big consumers, spending over $30 million on their grandchildren each year.

Sharing good news and sage advice with old friends is a formula that never gets old. What sets this shower apart from the others is that it's not about providing for baby's immediate needs. If Grandpa loves books, ask guests to start a "Lifetime of Reading" library. If Grandma is a fashionista, create a "dress-up" trunk. To create this event, you simply need to gather friends, family, or coworkers and have them bring equal parts of common sense, babysitting tips, and creativity.

Setting Up at Home

An at-home setting is a great backdrop for this type of shower. It allows for easy conversations, comfortable entertaining, and minimal preparation. As with all at-home parties, there are a few things to consider before you commit to opening your living room to guests. Your home will work for the Grandparents' Shower if:

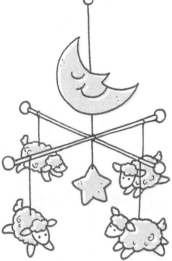

- ✓ **You have enough space to seat all guests.** If you don't have enough chairs, consider borrowing or renting them.
- ✓ **You have a way to cook or heat food for a crowd.** A standard oven, a microwave, or a barbeque grill can all be pressed into service, depending on your menu.
- ✓ **You have an area to serve food.** Buffet-style service can be set up on the dining room table, a kitchen counter, or an outdoor patio table.

Setting Up Away from Home

The best news about this shower is that you can have it anywhere. The Grandparents' Shower can make its home at the local bowling alley, the bocce ball courts, your favorite pizza palace, or a local steak house. Since the key ingredients are the same—good friends, good food, and good advice—it can be paired with another social activity, your monthly book club meeting, your gourmet cooking group, the bunco/poker-night group, or the tennis team. Some other alternative venues for the Grandparents' Shower include: golf course, tennis or athletic club, country club, park, or restaurant.

Menu Ideas

If you're having this shower in your home, keep the menu simple. This menu is easy to make and easy to serve. It can be made two days ahead, and it actually tastes better—the flavors have a chance to come together. This meal infuses your kitchen with the warm and inviting smells that remind you of Sunday suppers in Grandma's kitchen. This menu will work with all the party ideas in this chapter. To set up this one-pot meal, serve stew directly from the pot or ladle into bowls.

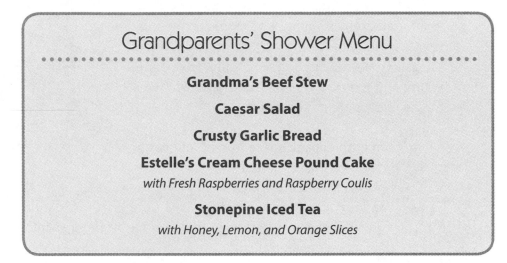

Grandparents' Shower Menu

Grandma's Beef Stew

Caesar Salad

Crusty Garlic Bread

Estelle's Cream Cheese Pound Cake
with Fresh Raspberries and Raspberry Coulis

Stonepine Iced Tea
with Honey, Lemon, and Orange Slices

Regardless of the specific theme you choose for the Grandparents' Shower, a simple, homey meal is mandatory. The beauty of the main course, Grandma's Beef Stew, is that it can be made ahead, can be reheated in one pot, and has universal appeal—not too spicy, yet full of flavor. The classic Caesar salad compliments the flavors perfectly. And as for dessert, what could beat the aroma of freshly baked chocolate pound cake!

Invitation Ideas

The invitation is often the first notice your guests will receive about your event. You can create invitations from all kinds of materials, but remember, this is your chance to express yourself, and most of all, have some fun! If you are planning to mail invitations, any blank card or specialty paper can become an invitation by simply printing a page from your computer. Use the wording below as a guide, but remember to convey a sense of fun about this upcoming event.

Include all the information you want your guests to know before they arrive at your event. You may want to use a traditional invitation wording like: You're invited to a Grandparents' Shower to celebrate the birth of a new set of grandparents! Come help Grandma and Grandpa get ready for this momentous occasion! Then include the other important information such as

"We're building a book collection for the grandbaby—bring your favorite children's book" (or movie, song, etc.).

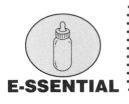

E-SSENTIAL

Paper invitations are available online at these Web sites: *www.tiny prints.com, www.simplytoimpress.com*. Or here is a sampling of sites that offer e-mail invitations: *www.sendomatic.com, www.evite.com, www.clickz.com*.

E-mail invitations should contain the same information as the snail mail invitation. You can send this in a standard e-mail or you can use one of the many electronic invitation sites now available. If you choose this option, make sure that all the invited guests have regular, daily access to a computer and e-mail account. If you don't have e-mail addresses for all your guests, opt for a phone call or a mailed invite.

Music and Entertainment

Music is a vital component to set a mood for your party. If you know the musical tastes of your guests, load up the CD changer and let the lyrics carry you away. The goal in selecting music is to ramp up the energy without overwhelming the conversation volume.

Depending on your budget, you may also decide to include some type of entertainment at your party. Musicians and entertainers can be contracted through a talent agency in your local area. Keep in mind that it is probably not necessary to hire a comedian, dancer, or the like—your guests will enjoy the opportunity to connect or reconnect with each other. If you feel that you would like to include some form of entertainment, consider hiring a guitarist to provide an element of live music. If you have a piano, hire someone to play it, and perhaps encourage guests to engage in a sing-a-long.

| THEME IDEA 1 | *Baby Libris—Start a Children's Book Collection* |

This shower theme is perfect for the grandparents who love books and all things literary. Encourage guests to give their favorite book from childhood or one recommended for young readers. A personalized inscription turns a storybook into a lasting keepsake.

Color Palette and Decor

For this shower, try working with three colors—black and white and *read* (red) all over. You can use black and white polka-dot or check linens and red or black napkins. White dishes add an uncluttered touch to this literary décor. Red roses, tulips, or carnations will add a punch of color to the table. Hot Tamales or Red Hots in clear mason jars, jelly jars, or wine glasses dot the serving table, interspersed with stacks of books wrapped in white butcher paper or newspaper. Use red licorice laces to tie napkins and flatware together.

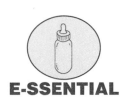

E-SSENTIAL

Restaurant supply stores are a treasure trove for the at-home hostess. Here you can find simple white plates for $1 per piece, or restaurant-quality stemware for $1.50 each. Flatware and linens are also available at a significant discount. Discount department stores also offer some other excellent items at bargain prices. Look in the phone book or on the Web for your local supplier.

Invitation Ideas and Script

Create your own version of a library checkout card using manila card-stock and a date stamp. Use your computer to recreate the columns or simply line them on with a ruler and black ink. Use the baby family name as the library name, with the hosting family's home as the branch.

Title: Baby Hanes
Authors: Tiffany and Thomas Hanes
Editors: "Nana" and "Papa" Hanes
Due Date: August 3rd
Come celebrate the release of this first edition
With a book "signing."
Friday, July 7th at 7:00 P.M.
Dinner at Hanes Library Building
Bring a favorite child's book and write in your good wishes.
Call the head librarian for more information!

The Perfect Game or Activity

"Name That Rhyme" game. Guests try to name that nursery rhyme with only a few words as the clue. For this game you will need:

✓ A nursery-rhyme book (*Classic Nursery Rhymes* by Paige Weber is a good one)
✓ A small pad of paper (one for each guest)
✓ Pens and paper (one for each guest)
✓ Rhyme quiz and answer sheet

Before the party begins, select phrases from the nursery-rhymes book. Choose two snippets per person for as many people as you expect (e.g., write thirty if you expect fifteen people). Create an answer sheet for yourself. Give all your guests a sheet of paper and a pen. Read the line aloud, as in "The sheep's in the meadow." Each guest must write the title of the rhyme from which the line is derived on their paper. Repeat until you've used all the rhyme snippets. Now go back and check the answers. Whoever has the most correct is the winner.

Variations on this game could include using lines from classic children's literature, movies, or songs.

Gifts That Work with This Theme

One of the best things about the Grandparents' Shower is that the gifts can be more whimsical or more unusual. In this case, guests are asked to give baby a book. The result will be an instant library. The books can be geared toward infants and toddlers or include books for baby's adolescence and young-adult years.

Other book-related ideas include:

✓ Personalized books with grandchild's name
✓ Bookends
✓ Baby scrap and photo book
✓ Bookcase (this would also be a great group gift)
✓ Rocking chair: perfect to rock and be read to!
✓ Tell-Me-a-Story Tape—a story you record on tape or CD (also a terrific activity at the shower—if you are techno-savvy)

Favors

Everybody likes to go home with a present, even a grandparent. These favors don't have to be baby related, and they don't have to break the bank.

✓ **Customized crossword puzzles.** There are Web sites that can create them while you wait, and others that take your order (see Appendix A).
✓ **Bookmarks or bookplates.** These can be simple, crafty creations or polished and customized. The Web offers dozens of sites to order from, such as *www.myownlabels.com, www.stationerystudio.com,* or you can create your own. Use the same style and art from the shower invitation to carry out the theme.

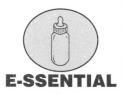

E-SSENTIAL

Some good group grandparents gifts include: a savings bond to start a college fund, a personalized piggy bank (filled, of course!), travel expenses for the out-of-town grandparents to visit the baby, new suitcase filled with baby essentials for impending visits to Grandma's house, or a crib for stays at grandparents' house.

THEME IDEA 2 *Save a Bundle Shower*

Whether the family is spread out across the country or right around the corner, chances are that the new grandbaby will be visiting grandma and grandpa. This shower is the perfect solution: Guests (and fellow grandparents) can recycle baby essentials like cribs, strollers, Pack 'n Plays, and the myriad clothes and other items that these small bundles seem to require.

Color Palette

Brown, black, and aluminum (shiny or matte) make a great combination for this recycling theme.

Carry out this theme by recycling or reinventing items you already have around the house. Cover your main table with a white or neutral tablecloth, then use burlap or brown parcel paper as a runner. Use brown lunch bags, rolled down half way and lined with tissue, to hold popcorn and movie candy for the activity. White dishes and twine-tied flatware/napkin bundles can become place cards with the addition of a shipping label, available at office supply stores. Use large tomato cans as recycled containers for your flowered centerpieces. Wash cans and fill with fresh basil, thyme, dill, parsley, and flowers. Labels can remain if you like them or be removed to reveal the aluminum—a more industrial look. Intersperse centerpieces with votive candles—or use cupcake pans to hold the votives.

Invitation Ideas and Script

Use a brown paper bag as the base for this invitation. Use rubber stamps (i.e. FRAGILE, RECYCLE, etc.) to decorate the bags. Print the invitations from your computer and glue to a cardboard base or write information directly on the bag using a black sharpie.

Recycling Project in Full Swing!
Joni and Lloyd are going to be Grandparents
And we're going to rejoice, recycle
And save a bundle on baby equipment!
Join us on Friday, October 22nd for dinner and movies!
Bring a gently used piece of baby equipment and your
favorite "baby" movie scene.
Prizes will be given for the best revisited scene.
R.S.V.P. to Lanie by October 5th

The Perfect Game or Activity

A binky, another name for a pacifier, is used to create a shower version of the four-star movie-rating system. One binky is poor, two binkies means average, three binkies means good, and four binkies means excellent. Use the four-binky scale to rate your favorite scene from a baby-related movie. On the invitation, ask guests to bring a two-minute clip from their favorite movie, preferably about babies or children; some examples are *Three Men and a Baby*, *Baby Boom*, *Look Who's Talking*, and *Parenthood*. Each guest presents his or her movie clip and the rest vote in various categories—funniest, most poignant, best acting, best delivery, and so on. See Appendix C for how to make a binky rating sheet. The person whose clip receives the highest binky rating wins.

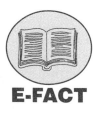

E-FACT

My Granny's Purse by P. H. Hanson is a delightful board book that is shaped like a purse and opens to reveal a collection of "mementos and magic." Also available is *My Grandpa's Briefcase* by the same author. Both books are surefire hits for the new Grandma and Grandpa.

Gifts That Work with This Theme

Anything on the Nursery Essentials list (see Chapter 8) that is in good condition, such as strollers, play saucers, high chairs, bassinettes, changing tables, toys, books, mobiles, and the like, might be a good gift. Used items should be wiped with a safe disinfecting solution, and changing pads and mattress pads or covers should be replaced. Guests and hostesses should also remember that Federal Safety Standards have changed significantly over the past fifty years. Cribs, playpens, strollers, car seats, even toys and clothing are manufactured under stricter guidelines.

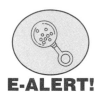

E-ALERT!

Federal Standards for baby equipment and baby-related products have changed. When recycling equipment, check manufacturing dates before using. Cribs should be manufactured during or after September 1986. (Older cribs have wider spaces between bars, now considered a danger.) Playpens should be made after 1976, and strollers should be manufactured after 1985.

The Essential Grandparents' Home Away from Home should have:

✓ Car seat (Current laws require children under forty-five pounds to be in a car seat—that's most four-year-olds.)
✓ Collapsible stroller
✓ High chair or booster seat
✓ Changing area with diapers, wipes, pad or towel, and trash can with liner and lid
✓ Bibs and burp cloths
✓ Blankets
✓ Towels and washcloths
✓ Baby monitor (optional)
✓ Dishwasher cages for baby items—spoons, bottle nipples, etc.

✓ Formula, baby food, cereal, juice
✓ Baby Medical Kit: thermometer, bulb syringe, nail clippers, infant Tylenol and dropper
✓ Soaps, shampoo, baby detergent
✓ Smoke detector

Favors

Candy favor bags filled with nostalgic candies (Necco Wafers, Mary Janes, Dots). To make these you will need:

✓ Cellophane bags (one per guest) 4" × 8½"
✓ ½ cup candy assortment per bag
✓ Cardstock labels, 4" × 6" (to be folded in half to 4" × 3")
✓ Decorative stickers that match the theme
✓ Stapler

1. Fill bags with candy.
2. Decorate labels and fold in half.
3. Fold down top of bag and staple label on each corner.

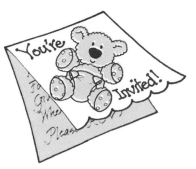

Chapter 13

Broadway Baby Shower: For Drama Buffs and Drama Queens

IF THE MOM-TO-BE knows the entire score from *Hairspray*, *Rent*, or *Phantom of the Opera*, she'll sing the praises of the Broadway Baby Shower. For lovers of the dramatic arts, what could be more fun? The beauty of planning a Broadway Baby Shower is its versatility. Revive an old classic musical like *Pajama Game* or *Carousel* and build your theme around the title, tone, or time frame. Use a show title with a twist—Avenue Poo (*Avenue Q*), Greased (*Grease*), or *The Producers* (perfect as is).

Who Can Use This Theme

When your shower audience consists of extroverts and lovers of arts, a Broadway Baby theme is just the ticket. The shower will work as well for couples as it will for a singles mix or girlfriends. Remember when compiling the guest list to include "actors," and "audience members"; after all, someone has to watch, admire, and applaud the performers! Stage mothers (and fathers) are also a great addition to the party cast. The theme would also work for families with children—especially if you focused the theme on children's plays or musicals.

The versatility of this theme is part of its wide appeal—you can focus on musicals from the 1950s or '60s or limit it to current Broadway productions. You can pay homage to Tony Award–winning shows or attend a local theater production. The theme can be adapted to any age group or musical taste.

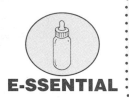

E-SSENTIAL

Carry out the Broadway theme by decorating with reproduction theater posters and playbills available at the Tony Shop. You can also find the Tony Awards Songbook and scripts of lost Broadway productions, so your guests can sing or act along. See Appendix A for more information.

Setting Up at Home

Setting the stage for your Broadway Baby Shower at home can be as simple an undertaking as your talents and your living room will allow. You will need a stage area if you are planning to play charades, encourage a sing-a-long, or have guests perform a scene from a play. Adjustable lighting can help to set a theater mood, but it doesn't have to be elaborate—twinkle lights can do the trick or up-lights, like the ones used to highlight plants, can be pressed into service. A sound system is a must, both as a backdrop to the party and to assist in any performance piece. If your budget and setting can support it, consider hiring a musician, particularly a piano or guitar player to make the sing-a-long a reality. Curtains, the theater-type, can add to the drama by providing the much-needed element of shock and surprise when they are opened. If your home has a natural stage, consider setting up a curtain. Theater props are available for purchase or rental through some local theater companies and some high schools with larger performance departments.

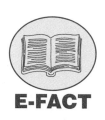

E-FACT

Fondue pots have come a long way since the 1970s; they are available in many sizes, styles, and finishes (no more harvest gold or avocado). They come in electric and flame-top styles (these require the use of a burner with gel or solid fuel). Use traditional metal fondue forks or long bamboo skewers to dip each tasty morsel.

Setting Up Away from Home

The nation abounds with old theaters, many available for parties. If your shower will include a performance element, consider renting a theater to stage the party. Serve concession-style food or theme the food to compliment the title of the shower; for example, if you choose Flower Drum Song, serve Chinese food or set up dim sum stations.

Of course, it is not a necessity to have guests performing at the shower; after all it's a baby shower—the stars are mother- and baby-to-be. Besides, theater buffs will enjoy any type of theater experience, so consider planning the shower around a local production of a favorite show. Keep in mind travel time, cost per ticket, and length of shower (pregnant women cannot sit for long periods without a stretch and a ladies room).

Menu Ideas and Options

If you're fond of fondue, you will give this fun and delicious menu a standing ovation. The beauty of this meal is the interactive element that comes with trying different combinations of dippers and dips. The classic cheese recipe can serve as an appetizer or, with the addition of sausage and chopped chicken, can become a main course. The dessert fondues, both chocolate and creamy caramel, are a grand finale to an evening that celebrates a new baby, old friendships, and Broadway music.

Broadway Baby Shower Menu

A Classic Cheese Fondue

Served with a Variety of Breads (Pumpernickel, Rye, Bagel Chunks, Soft Pretzels, Sourdough, or French Bread), Blanched Cauliflower, Broccoli, Mushrooms, and Potatoes, crisp Apples, and Cooked Meats and Sausages

A Classic Chocolate Fondue and a Classic Caramel Fondue

Served with an Assortment of "Dippers," Like Strawberries, Pineapple, Pears, Bing Cherries, Bananas, Dried Apricots, Mango, Papaya, Yellow Cake, Angel Cake, Lady Fingers, Brownies, Snickers, Gummy Bears, Lorna Doones, Marshmallows, Rice Krispy Treats, Pretzels, and Graham Crackers

---

Guests will enjoy the two dipping choices for this dessert fondue station. Arrange dippers at various heights and in unusual open containers—try apothecary-style jars, pedestal bowls, and trays. As a final touch, serve chocolate jimmies, pink or blue sprinkles, and chopped pistachios and almonds.

Invitation Ideas and Script

For this invitation, a reproduction of a theatre ticket fits the bill. This invitation can be created on your computer if you have the software for graphic arts; however, there are a number of places online that offer ticket-style invitations with a quick turn-around time and for a nominal charge.

Come sing the lullaby of Broadway for
Ken and Jen's Broadway Baby
at a Shower and Command Performance
Saturday, April 13th

| **Mamma Mia:** *A Shower and Musical Review for Couples*

Mamma Mia is a shower tribute to rock musicals. Inspired by shows like *Hair, Jesus Christ Superstar, Grease,* and *Tommy,* this party will be as toe-tapping as the musicals that inspired it are!

Color Palette and Decor

Black. Neon Brights. Heavy Metal. Faded denim. You get the vibe! Anything goes when rock and disco collide. This theme breaks the rules. Now's your chance to do the same. Mix denim and tattoos, black lace and spikes, or platforms and flower power to create the mood. Reproduction show posters can serve as art or table runners. Short glass cylinders filled with snapped Glo-sticks in neon colors will provide a theatrical flourish. Dangle inflatable instruments from ribbons on chairs or banisters. Change the light bulbs in the party room to blue—this casts a vintage nightclub vibe over your party. And don't forget the disco ball!

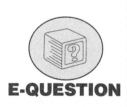

E-QUESTION

What about costumes?
Part of the drama of the theater is the costume. The costume helps the actors create their characters and lets the audience understand the actor's role. There are costume rental shops all over, but if your town doesn't have one, head to the secondhand store and bring your imagination. Hats, belts, gloves, capes, coats, neckties, scarves, and jewelry can help guests get into character.

The Perfect Game or Activity

The name of the game is Karaoke-Go-Round. Turn your living room into a recording studio and play your own version of *American Idol.* Tell guests ahead of time that karaoke will be encouraged! You will need:

- ✓ Karaoke system or magic microphone
- ✓ Karaoke CD, children's songs, music from the 1950s or '60s, Broadway—whatever you think your group will enjoy the most
- ✓ Stage area, as simple as cleared floor space (4' × 6' is adequate) or with a riser, backdrop, lights, and optional disco ball

Gifts That Work with This Theme

A "Musical Table" that holds four percussion instruments or a basket of instruments from the local toy store are perfect for the budding music prodigy (*www.backtobasicstoys.com*).

Other gift ideas include:

- ✓ Music classes for babies and adults
- ✓ Rock Star Baby T-shirts (*www.rockstarbaby.com*)
- ✓ Personalized CDs—featuring music that has baby's name in it (*www.mymusiccd.com, www.aspecialgift.com, www.bamababiesandbirthdays.com*)
- ✓ Musical videos for babies (e.g., The Wiggles, Blues Clues, PBS Kids)
- ✓ For the superambitious—ask the musically inclined guests to bring their instruments and stage a jam session. Create a recording of this once-in-a-lifetime event!

Favors

A custom CD with a mix of songs from your favorite Broadway shows is relatively easy to make, and it will have guests singing in the shower or commuter lane. Most CDs hold about eighteen to twenty songs. Labels can be customized, and the carrying case can be a copy of the invitation art. See *www.everydayeventplanner.com* for CD case art.

Also, consider these other favor ideas:

- ✓ Children's music CD
- ✓ Glo-necklaces
- ✓ Magic microphones
- ✓ Kazoos

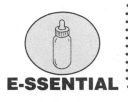

THEME IDEA 2 | **Hello Dolly!** *Welcoming the Newest Star*

Say "Hello, Dolly!" with a party styled in the tradition of grand entrances much like the new baby girl will make. This theme celebrates the theatrical with feather boa'd décor and ostrich plumes straight out of Dolly Levi's costume closet. Enormous Victorian hats, bouquets of red and pink roses, and yards of pearls will help to carry out the essence of this theme. An essential part of the party fun will be the creation of a costume trunk befitting the modern-day theater diva.

Color Palette and Decor

Since this version of the Broadway Baby Shower is more appropriate for a group of women who are marking the arrival of a new baby girl, the mix of leopard-print and red to hot-pink roses (oranges or paler pinks will also work) is girlie and theatrical—the perfect backdrop for fun. Display the dress-up trunk in a prominent place so guests can drop their dress-up items in as they arrive. Use your sterling silver or buy coordinated paperware in a wild leopard print. If you have silver metal candlesticks or candelabras, drape them in strands of dime-store pearls. Bouquets of ostrich feathers can alternate with clusters of colorful roses. Take out your teddy bear collection and dress up several to join the festivities as centerpieces or on the serving table. Use expandable dime-store rings as napkin holders.

The Perfect Game and Activity

You can incorporate this easy game, Who Has the Heaviest Purse? into the party schedule. A gag gift—candy lipstick or necklace, a coin purse, or certificate of the winner's status as "Heaviest-Purse Holder" is all that is needed as a prize.

This game is simple and takes absolutely no skill. It does require a kitchen or bathroom scale. Simply weigh each woman's purse. It's unbelievable how much women carry around. The guest with the heaviest purse wins.

Or you could try Broadway Baby Charades, a game that involves acting out words or phrases in pantomime to members of an audience who are divided into teams. The team who guesses correctly first gets a point, and the team with the most points wins.

To play you will need: a stopwatch or watch, a paper and pen to keep score, blank paper strips with words or phrases, and two baskets for the slips. Play time should be forty-five minutes to one hour.

1. Prepare a charade slip for each guest with a phrase, production title (e.g., *Man of La Mancha*), song title, character, or theater phrase that they could act out.
2. Form two teams of equal size and give each team member the charade slips.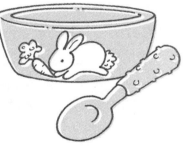
3. Teach standard charade gestures and hand signals.
4. Toss a coin to determine which team goes first. Allow a few moments for the teams to retreat to strategize and create their phrases.
5. Set the timer for three minutes and let the first person act out her phrase in gestures without speaking. Any talking by the actor means disqualification, and play reverts to the other team.
6. The opposite team has to shout out their guesses, and the actor and his team have to acknowledge any correct guess.
7. If the team does not guess the phrase in the allotted time, they lose the round.
8. Play until everyone on both teams has had a chance to be an actor. The team with the most points wins.

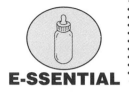

E-SSENTIAL

Gifts That Work with This Theme

The hostess(es) may want to provide a trunk as the container for the contents to come. The trunk can be as elaborate as an antique steamer trunk or as simple as a cardboard storage box. Many container stores carry printed boxes with lids or closet organizers that could also be used to store precious dress-up items.

The best part about this gift is that there is no limit to how silly or outlandish the items are, or how many there are. More is better! Here are some ideas and suggestions:

- ✓ **Feather boas.** They come in every color.
- ✓ **Gloves.** Whether white, sequined, long, fingerless, wooly, colorful, lacey—anything goes.
- ✓ **Hats.** Everything from simple berets to elaborate bonnets will work.
- ✓ **Scarves.** Perfect in all sizes, shapes, and fabrics.
- ✓ **Jewelry.** Long strands of beads, rings, clip earrings, and bracelets, especially jingly ones. For safety's sake, avoid anything with jagged edges; sharp, pointy pins; or parts or loose stones.
- ✓ **Dresses.** Old prom dresses are a little girl's dream. Anything sparkly, bright, and out-of-fashion is perfect for the trunk.
- ✓ **Shoes.** High heels, sling-backs, sandals, dance shoes—all are perfect for the trunk. Most toy stores now carry "high heels" in children's sizes.
- ✓ **Costumes.** Halloween costumes of every kind will find a good home in the dress-up box.
- ✓ **Wigs.** New or well-cleaned (and disinfected) wigs are always a hit, especially as children get older.

Be sure to have large two-gallon zip-top storage bags and tissue available to wrap and store each item.

Favors

What lady doesn't covet a new purse? These "flower-power" felt purses give Victorian style to today's haute mammas. Fill these lovely bags with a few chocolates, rose-petal tea, or candied violets. The bags, which come in an assortment of styles and colors, will add a humorous and decorative touch wherever you display them.

| THEME IDEA 3 | *Baby Grand: A Piano-Bar Sing-Along Shower* |

From singing in the shower to singing at the shower, this rendition of Broadway Baby will be the talk of the town. It's musically jam-packed, since guests will be instructed to come prepared to sing for their supper. Don't let stage fright limit the guest list—the performance-challenged can take on other roles, like master of ceremonies, stage manager, or props coordinator. All you need to make this shower happen is a pregnant mommy and a piano player—either friend or for hire. Best of all, the party can be modified to work for adults or families with children simply by changing the time, tweaking the menu, and adjusting the song selections.

Color Palette and Decor

For this shower, the decorating palette is more about drama than color. Deep jewel tones of ruby crimson, emerald green, sapphire blue, and amethyst purple will provide a stunning backdrop for this performance. Add some sparkle with gold, copper, or silver—but not all three—it's too distracting. Candelabras, piano shawls, and velvet runners add richness and sparkle to the décor, making it a sophisticated adult evening soiree. Sheet-music coasters, piano-key napkins, and a note-worthy martini or mamatini (see Chapter 5), and you've got yourself a swanky shower. If your audience is on the younger side, change up the colors by going primary—red, green, blue, and purple to make it more kid-friendly. A shimmer curtain, available at many craft or party stores, is a great backdrop for a family sing-along.

Add tambourines, maracas, and bells to allow all the "kids" to participate, even if they are too shy to act or sing.

The Perfect Game or Activity

Make your guests sing for their supper! In order to make this shower the best it can be, you will need to do some extra coordinating before the guests arrive. Tell guests what you will have available for them to use, for example, a piano player, a piano, a drum set, a hand-held microphone. Let guests know what they will need to bring—props, sheet music, costumes, and so on, when you send out the invitations. Ask guests to R.S.V.P. with their performance piece so the musicians can prepare. A response phone call or e-mail is essential to give you a firm number for actors and audience—you don't want to be short chairs or seating. If you have a master of ceremonies, work out the order of acts in advance with him or her. It takes a little foresight and planning to make the evening flow more smoothly. Intersperse up-beat songs and routines with quieter ones to keep things moving. The piano player can invite the audience to sing along with old standbys between acts.

On shower day, allow enough time (usually about a half hour) beforehand for the "artistes" to bring in and set up any special equipment they will need. Most singers don't like to perform on a full stomach, so the show should be the first act. As an added and interesting "Ta-Da," have each entertainer spotlight their gift by presenting it to the mom-to-be as they conclude their number. Applause, applause, and dinner is served. Plan to open gifts during coffee after the meal.

Gifts That Work with This Theme

As with the other Broadway-themed showers, gifts that play on the new parents' musical interests are perfect. Here are some other ideas that will work with this theme:

- ✓ Baby-sized baby grand piano
- ✓ Baby chandelier
- ✓ Broadway onesies

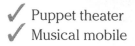 Puppet theater
 Musical mobile

Favors

It's a theater tradition to give flowers to the actors after the show. This favor is a rose with a flavor; they are made from chocolate kisses! These take-aways are easy to make (even preteens can help put them together), and they can serve as décor—display them in a cut-crystal vase on the piano. "Kiss" each guest as they make their curtain call for the evening. Make a special bouquet to send home with the real star of the show—the mommy-to-be.

For instructions on how to make these candy rose favors, check out *www.everydayeventplanner.com.*

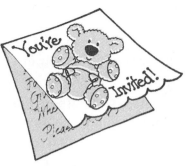

Chapter 14

Jack and Jill Showers for Couples

THERE WAS A TIME when the only role a father seemed to have in the birthing of the baby was that of the comical, bumbling, mildly distraught man who got mom to the hospital and then paced the halls. Those days are long gone. In their place are competent men who share in the experiences and responsibilities of child rearing. This chapter offers shower opportunities made for sharing with the boys.

Who Can Use This Theme

These parties are designed for couples and friends who want to celebrate the joy of a new life with both the new mom and the new dad. The party-loving guests need have no fear of arriving at a high tea and crumpets soiree. Themes are energetic, activity driven, guy-friendly, loud, and totally free of baby trivia and other itty-bitty infant concerns like diaper rash and breast feeding. In this chapter, you will find three very different party themes: "Diapers Wild!," a poker party and tournament; "Lucky Strike Bowling Night;" and the "LaMaze–LeMans Road Rally," a scavenger hunt by car. As a result, they are being presented with their own menu, activity, and invitation options. If you are intrigued by the concepts, but daunted by the prospect of planning these showers, consider hiring a professional. For a fee, a casino company can arrive at your venue with everything you will need to set up a high-rollers poker tournament—from chips to tables to dealers. Many bowling alleys have party coordinators on-site who will organize lanes, teams, and even provide food. Across the nation, there are car clubs and private businesses who set up, map out, and manage road rallies. See Appendix A for more information.

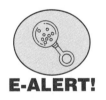

E-ALERT!

You will not see six-foot sandwich loaves in your grocery store, but you can order them through any bread baker. Allow several days to a week to receive the order and be sure to clear out a space in the back of the car to accommodate its ride home.

THEME IDEA 1 | *Diapers Wild! A Poker Party and Shower*

Here's a couples shower idea that will certainly pack a full house—a Poker Tournament! Bring Las Vegas-style poker right into your living room. This is definitely not your mother's baby shower. Keep a few traditions—like betting on baby's birth date and weight, passing out cigars (bubblegum, of course), and opening presents.

Invitation Ideas and Script

There are lots of ready-made poker-party invitation options available nearly everywhere. Have some fun when wording the invitation by using poker terminology.

Diapers Wild! A Jack and Jill Poker Tournament
We're celebrating Baby Smith's arrival and this is no bluff
Ante up—We've got dealers and diapers in spades
You may know how to hold 'em, we'll show you how to fold 'em
Saturday, April 4th at 7 P.M.
It will be a full house, be here for the big finish!

Menu Ideas and Options

When men are on the guest list, think hearty menu. One surefire hit is the classic sub sandwich. A six-foot Italian submarine sandwich (which serves up to thirty people) will be the star of the buffet table. Pair it up with potato salad, potato chips, coleslaw, or a green salad, and then serve sandwiches for dessert—ice-cream sandwiches (either store-bought or handmade with chocolate-chip cookies, mmmmm), of course!

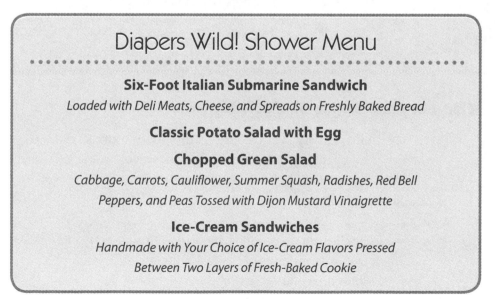

Diapers Wild! Shower Menu

Six-Foot Italian Submarine Sandwich
Loaded with Deli Meats, Cheese, and Spreads on Freshly Baked Bread

Classic Potato Salad with Egg

Chopped Green Salad
Cabbage, Carrots, Cauliflower, Summer Squash, Radishes, Red Bell Peppers, and Peas Tossed with Dijon Mustard Vinaigrette

Ice-Cream Sandwiches
Handmade with Your Choice of Ice-Cream Flavors Pressed Between Two Layers of Fresh-Baked Cookie

Color Palette and Décor

Poker night conjures up the image of green-felt table tops, red and black poker chips, and colorful decks of playing cards. To create this look in your home, start with a roll of green felt to use as tablecloths for the playing tables and food table. Green plastic or paper will also work.

Although the giant sub sandwich is almost décor enough, give the table a poker face with a few casino-esque touches. Arrange clusters of red carnations and baby's breath tucked into die-cut gift bags shaped like a hand of playing cards (it will be your secret that they are in small plastic containers hidden from view). Alternate with pots of marigolds in the same bags to punch up the color. Deck the table with chocolate poker chips, gold coins, play money, and loose cards. String Christmas-style lights around or take the lights over the top with strands of lighted red dice (see Appendix A). Bowls of peanuts, pretzels, and red and black licorice will keep players holding, not folding.

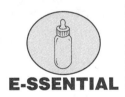

E-SSENTIAL

Customized playing cards are easy to order and affordable, and they make great party favors and remembrances that can actually be used. Order them with a phrase like "Diapers Wild!" or "Baby Needs New Shoes!" with baby's name and the shower date, or send in a photo or other artwork to be printed on the back of each card.

The Perfect Game or Activity

The main activity for this party is the poker tournament. For seasoned players, a tournament can take all night; however, a quick-fire tourney can be done in about an hour. To set up a poker tournament for up to thirty people, you will need:

✓ Poker Tournament Rules and Procedures (see Appendix A)
✓ Ten standard decks of cards, unopened
✓ Poker chips in three colors
✓ Poker tables to seat six to eight comfortably

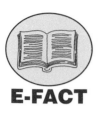

E-FACT

Here are the common poker chip colors and point values: Red = 5, Green = 25, Black = 100, Purple = 500, and Yellow = 1,000—you only need three colors of chips for a standard at-home game—red, green, and black. If you are using the three colors, start each player with 1,000 points worth of chips, broken down as follows: twenty red, twenty green, and four black.

There are a number of Web sites and books that give detailed instructions for setting up home tournaments. It is not necessary to choose a complicated plan—remember, it's a game. Stick with the standard poker rules, (this is no time to get fancy) and keep a copy of the rules at each table for quick reference. Rule books are available for download from the U.S. Poker Web site.

Another fun activity is taking a gamble on guessing when baby will be born. All you have to do is create this simple chart.

Betting on Baby Chart:

1. Draw a grid with enough squares to accommodate a guess from each party guest. For example: If you have thirty guests, draw a grid five squares across and six squares down.
2. Across the top, label each column with a date starting a day or two before the baby's due date and ending a day or two after the due date.
3. Down the left side, label each row with a baby weight in pounds and ounces. (You can also estimate time of arrival if your group prefers.)
4. Each guest chooses a square that represents the date and weight that they want to "bet" on. Write in the guest's name and phone number or e-mail address.
5. Notify the winner when the big day arrives!

Gifts That Work with This Theme

This kind of shower is a perfect opportunity for guests to go in on a group gift. Consider pooling your resources and purchasing big-ticket items like:

✓ A jogging stroller
✓ Baby bike trailer
✓ Baby furniture—a changing table or rocking chair

Favors

No poker tournament would be complete without the dealer visor. Order these green plastic visors and customize them the with theme "Diapers Wild!" on a laser-printed label or with puff paints. A sweet favor that won't be a gamble is the Sin City Sucker—a dice-shaped lollipop in flavors like Pina Co*Slot*a, Orange You Lucky, Cherry Cherry Cherry, and Grape of Spades (see Appendix A).

THEME IDEA 2 | *Lucky Strike! From Bowling Pins to Diaper Pins*

Take a step back in time with this party idea. If you haven't been bowling lately, there has been a renaissance in this sport. Alleys are updated and feature rock music, glow-in-the-dark graphics and pins, and neon signs. Many offer Extreme Bowling, Moonlight Bowling, and party deals that include use of lanes, shoe rental, and a party room for one and a half to two hours. Some packages also include food, and most places that offer food will not let you bring in your own.

You should plan on playing no more than two full games, which take about an hour. Depending on the size and skill level of your group, you may opt to play only one. Typically, four people play in each lane, which allows everyone enough bowling opportunities and keeps things moving. Leagues generally play late in the evening, so check with your local alley before setting a time for the shower.

Generally, you bowl first, then eat and open gifts. Award silly prizes and trophies to the players during the meal, and open gifts afterward. Another way to stage this shower is to have guests meet at the bowling alley, bowl a match, then return to your home for the eating and gift opening.

Invitation Ideas and Script

This bowling-shoe-shaped invitation could be the right fit for your couple's baby shower. Use a bowling invitation design or search clipart on the Web for a retro-look design. Print these from your computer, two on a page, pink the edges with pinking shears, and mount on heavy cardstock.

Grab your bowling shoes
And join us for
Lucky Strike!
As we celebrate
Diane and Steve's journey
From Bowling Pins to Diaper Pins!
Sunday, June 15th at 4 o'clock
Pizza Dinner to follow at the Alley Oops! Café

Menu Ideas and Options

This is no time to get fancy or trendy. When at the bowling alley, eat what the regulars eat—bowling-alley fare. This includes pizza, nachos, baskets of French fries, burgers, and hot dogs.

If you are serving guests a meal back at your home after the bowling activity, carry the bowling glossary into the food.

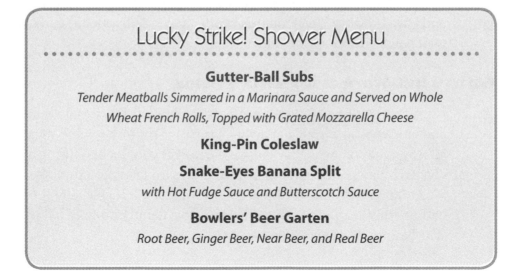

Lucky Strike! Shower Menu

Gutter-Ball Subs

Tender Meatballs Simmered in a Marinara Sauce and Served on Whole Wheat French Rolls, Topped with Grated Mozzarella Cheese

King-Pin Coleslaw

Snake-Eyes Banana Split

with Hot Fudge Sauce and Butterscotch Sauce

Bowlers' Beer Garten

Root Beer, Ginger Beer, Near Beer, and Real Beer

Color Palette and Décor

There's not much to decorate at this shower—if you have purchased a party package, the alley will supply tablecloths and paper goods. Bouquets of balloons can be brought in and are an easy way to provide quick setup and to say "Baby Bowler on Board."

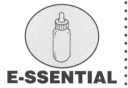

E-SSENTIAL

Bring your own appetizer cheese ball to the alley to get the party rolling. Purchase a premade cheese ball from the grocery store along with a bag of blue tortilla chips. Crush the chips into a coarse meal by placing them in a paper bag and hitting with a rolling pin. Roll the cheese into the crushed chips until all the cheese is completely covered. Use a melon baller to scoop out three "holes" in a triangle formation to resemble a bowling ball. Serve with crackers.

Setting up at home requires a little more planning. A bowling theme requires retro colors—turquoise, orangeade, Pepto-Bismol pink, and chartreuse in irregular, amoeba, and boomerang shapes are the order of the day. Bowl over friends with a toddler bowling kit. Set up pins (in some kits they look like bunnies, in others they are barnyard animals) in the center of the table. Fill clear glass fish bowls with Lucky Strike candy cigarettes and have bowls of "Ten Frame Popcorn," a blend of popcorn and chocolate malt balls—delicious for munching.

Gifts That Work with This Theme

A Bowling Bag Diaper Bag is a great gift idea. The classic bowling bag goes to work in a new capacity—for baby. These bags are inexpensive, kitschy, and practical; they can be ordered at your local bowling alley, purchased online, or even found at thrift stores and vintage clothing shops.

Or maybe a Baby Bowling T-shirt. A great gift, especially if mom and dad are in a bowling league. These cotton T-shirts proudly tell the world, "I'm Daddy's/Mommy's little bowler."

Favors

Since bowling is a team activity, consider giving guests a T-shirt that bears the shower theme. These can be ordered at a silk-screening shop (many athletic stores offer this service), or you can create your own iron-on transfer. There are a multitude of bowling-related Web sites that also offer bowling graphics that can be purchased. If you have divided guests into teams prior to the shower, order shirts in team colors to make play even easier.

And who doesn't love a trophy? Plan to award prizes in a variety of categories for this shower. Choose "Most Gutterballs," "Best Swing," "Lowest Points," in addition to the high-scorer prizes. Trophies come in all sizes and price ranges, but they are often coveted by tournament winners.

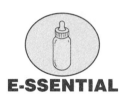

E-SSENTIAL

If T-shirts and trophies aren't your style, try giving crazy socks as a favor. Specialty socks are available online and in gift shops. Socks printed to look like bowling shoes or sneakers, socks with toes, even argyles would be a fun way to say thanks for coming.

THEME IDEA 3 | *The LaMaze–LeMans Car-Seat Rally*

A car rally may seem like an unlikely way to celebrate baby, but it can be an interesting and memorable way to help new parents celebrate with their friends. The invited group arrives at the rally starting point where they are given instructions about where to go, along with general directions for how to get there. Guests are teamed up in groups of four or six, depending on the size of the vehicle that will be making the trip, and then they drive from the start point to the end point as instructed in the route directions.

A road rally is not a race. Participants must follow all local and state traffic laws. They are completely legal, and they do not require any special permits. Along the route, signs are posted that give either further instructions, route alternates, or valuable information that will be needed to decode riddles or clues en route to the destination.

A successful rally requires mapping out a strategy and a road route, but it is well worth the extra effort. This shower is the party solution for car buffs and is a great way to get men involved with all the planning. What's more, they will be willing and excited participants.

Invitation Ideas and Script

The LaMaze-LeMans Road Rally requires an innovative invitation. For a full-throttle version, hot glue a Matchbox toy car on.

Hit the Road with us!
The LaMaze-LeMans
A Road-Rally Baby Shower to honor
Kate and Scott
And help them celebrate the newest member of their team!
Saturday, February 13th at 10 o'clock in the morning
We will stop for lunch at Jake's Pizza and be back by 4 P.M.
With plenty of pit stops along the way.

Menu Ideas and Options

Since dinner will be served at the destination, the only additional food that is needed for this party is the "One for the Road" snack pack. You can assemble individual backpacks or fanny packs and count them as favors, or you can pack a Styrofoam cooler for each car. Here are some popular snack items:

- ✓ Bottled water or flavored water
- ✓ Bottled or canned Frappacinos or other coffee-flavored drinks
- ✓ Travel mug with hot coffee (sippy cup optional)
- ✓ Rocky Road Trail Mix—nuts, marshmallows, and three kinds of chocolate chips
- ✓ NASCAR Pez dispenser and candies

Color Palette and Décor

Use the color palette straight from the road way—Stop-Sign Red, Caution-Light Yellow, Go Green, and Asphalt Black, mixed with checkered flags to carry your theme across the finish line. Road signs, caution tape, and colorful pennants should figure prominently in the day's décor. Give each car a pennant flag to tie to the antenna and mark their inclusion in the rally as they hit the road. Fill cellophane bags with snack mix and tie with bright-yellow caution tape. Be sure to have a checkered flag at the ready when guests arrive at the final pit stop.

Choosing the Rally Route and Perfect Destination

There are lots of organizations and car clubs that sponsor and create road rallies. Many have Web pages with route suggestions and rules. There are also books available on this subject. Remember to allow about eight weeks to plan and prepare for a road rally. To get you revved up about planning the LaMaze–LeMans Road Rally, there are some basic road rules:

✓ **Choose a finish destination.** Consider local eateries of interest—a famous hot dog stand, a local diner, a popular burger joint, or a happening sports bar. The destination should have ample parking and be able to accommodate the number of guests you will be bringing there to eat. You could also end at a beach or park and have guests pack a picnic lunch.

✓ **Select a starting point.** This should be within a few miles of the finish destination to facilitate getting guests back to their cars easily. It should have good parking, restroom facilities, and be easily accessible to roads and highways.

✓ **Determine a route.** Even though your starting and ending destinations may be reasonably close to each other, for the road rally you will be taking the scenic route to get there. The ride from point A to point B should be anywhere from ten to fifteen miles long, with three to five "pit stops" and lots of interesting things to see. Keep in mind that pregnant women require frequent bathroom breaks, so allow for a route that can accommodate this need.

✓ **Map the route, run the route, then map it again.** Once you have determined the roads to be traveled, prepare a map. Then drive the route yourself to double-check mileage, markers, and other considerations. Once you are satisfied that the route will work, finalize the map.

✓ **Label the route.** On rally day, you must put up signs and clues along the route to assist rally drivers in finding their destination. Print signs clearly and post securely in prominent areas. At each pit stop, offer a clue for where to find the next sign or a hint about the destination.

✓ **Prepare an information package.** Make sure every car has cell phone numbers and other vital information in case a car gets lost or other problems arise.

The Perfect Game or Activity

The rally may be all the activity you will need, but if there is lag time while waiting for guests to finish the rally, challenge friends to map out the shortest route to the hospital. Check routes on a GPS system or at Mapquest to determine the shortest distance between mom and delivery.

Gifts That Work with This Theme

When the theme is travel, baby equipment that makes traveling easier will get the checkered flag.

✓ **Car seat.** This is a great group gift. Federal law requires new parents to have a car seat before they leave the hospital with their new bundle of joy.

✓ **Baby backpack carrier.** Let baby be a backseat driver and see what Mom and Dad are up to.

✓ **Sheepskin car-seat covers.** Keep baby warm in winter and cool in summer.

✓ **Car seat accessories.** Toys that strap on to the seat tray, mirrors that allow mom and dad to see baby from the driver's seat, and sun shades that affix to windows to protect baby from burning rays are all much-needed items.

Favors

A memento of the big rally is all that is needed to say thanks for coming. Try ordering customized key rings or create a LaMaze–LeMans bumper sticker. Fanny packs or backpacks for the travel snacks also could be part of the favor packs.

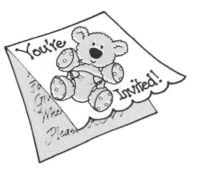

Chapter 15

Being Neighborly
Showers

GET TO KNOW the people in your community with these
neighborly party ideas. If you don't already know your
street or building mates, make use of a classic childhood
icon, the red wagon, fill it with munchies and drinks, and
take a walk around the "block" or down the hallway. It's
a great way to meet, greet, and make friends.

Who Can Use This Theme

The Red Wagon Showers (as they are commonly called) have been developed to work in a suburban setting, though they can be adapted to any friendly neighborhood. Enlist help from one and all to keep the affair on track; it will lighten the workload and increase the camaraderie on your block. The showers are designed to work whether it's a cook-it-together format or a progressive-dinner slant. Unlike many of the showers in this book, these showers will accommodate many planners and encourage friends and family to give gifts of time and helping hands, rather than presents of a more commercial nature.

The "Red Wagon" progressive-dinner shower puts mom on the move and spreads the task of planning and preparing around the neighborhood. The party moves from house to house, from appetizers to dessert, and the hostess at each house provides one course. In the "Red Wagon Food Challenge" baby shower, partygoers become the chefs, and they will cook up a dinner that incorporates a secret ingredient—baby food; while competing for the title of Whining Chef. Best of all, no purchased gifts are required; instead, the new mom receives neighborly offers of everything she could need after the birth of her baby—from babysitting to yard work to carpool duty. As a variation on other shower ideas, ask guests to bring a package of diapers to the shower of a friend then donate them to a local diaper drive.

THEME IDEA 1   Red Wagon Progressive Shower

A progressive dinner is a great way for neighbors to plan a shower together. The idea is this: Select three homes within walking distance of each other, have each home's hostess serve a dinner course, and then have guests move from house to house for the meal. Load the "Bar" in a red wagon, complete with soft drinks, beer, and ice, then move it with the party.

The first house should provide appetizers and cocktails, the second house dishes up a main course, and the final destination supplies dessert and coffee. This is also where gifts should be opened.

Setting It Up

For this party, planning together is a vital factor in making it a success. Start by getting together with other neighbors to determine who will host each phase and how many guests can be accommodated. In planning the menu, remember to coordinate cuisines; after all, some flavors just don't mix. Try going Italian—from antipasto to lasagna to tiramisu—or think Tex-Mex—from sangria to fajitas to sopaipillas.

The progressive dinner should be three to four hours long, which means an hour or less per house, including walking time. The evening's schedule might look like this:

✓ 7:00 P.M. Cocktails and Hors D'oeurves at Nancy and Bill's at 145 Main Street
✓ 7:45 P.M. Head to Dinner
✓ 8:00 P.M. Dinner at Sandy and Bob's, 158 Main St.
✓ 9:15 P.M. Head to Dessert and Presents
✓ 9:30 P.M. Dessert, Coffee, and Presents at Lulu and Kevin's, 175 Main St.

In this scenario, guests have ample time to get to the next location, and the opportunity to visit. If you live in a cul-de-sac, travel time may be shorter, but remember, it's not always that easy to get everybody moving.

Progressive Planning Tips:

✓ **Select foods that can be made ahead and quickly reheated when guests arrive.** The hostess for the next leg may need to leave a few minutes ahead of the group to get a jump on preparations; do not plan elaborate garnishes, sauces, or presentations—you won't have time.
✓ **Table and serving platters should be set and ready before the start time.** As the hostess, you will have only moments to get things from oven or refrigerator to table.
✓ **Extra beverages should be available at each location in addition to the portable Red Wagon bar.**

✓ **Stick to the schedule but don't rush guests.** Let everyone know what the timing is on the invitation. Post schedule and next location at each home so guests know what's coming.

✓ **Have a Plan B for getting the guest of honor from house to house if she is too pregnant to do so easily.**

Invitation Ideas and Script

This shower option also works well during the holiday season, when houses are dressed in their finery, and hostesses want to show them off.

There's gonna be a new kid on the block!
Roll out the welcome wagon
And join us for an All-American Progressive Baby Shower
To honor
Meredith, Nate and their bundle of joy
Sunday, May 18th at 7:00 in the evening
7:00 P.M. Cocktails and Hors D'oeurves at
Nancy and Bill's at 145 Main Street
8:00 P.M. Dinner at Sandy and Bob's, 158 Main Street
9:30 P.M. Dessert, Coffee and Presents at
Lulu and Kevin's, 175 Main Street

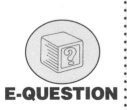

E-QUESTION

What can I do if my neighborhood won't work for a progressive dinner?
No neighborhood? No problem! Find a street in your business district or downtown area with a few local hot spots. Plan to stop first for cocktails and appetizers, then move on to the next location for the main course. The last stop should be the grand finale—coffee, dessert, and presents! Be sure to make reservations and wear comfortable shoes.

Menu Ideas and Options

Everyone will be excited about this barbeque menu. Load up a bright red wagon with bar fixings and keep it moving from house to house with the party.

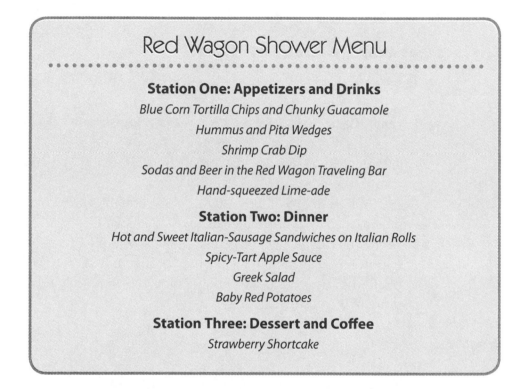

Red Wagon Shower Menu

Station One: Appetizers and Drinks

Blue Corn Tortilla Chips and Chunky Guacamole

Hummus and Pita Wedges

Shrimp Crab Dip

Sodas and Beer in the Red Wagon Traveling Bar

Hand-squeezed Lime-ade

Station Two: Dinner

Hot and Sweet Italian-Sausage Sandwiches on Italian Rolls

Spicy-Tart Apple Sauce

Greek Salad

Baby Red Potatoes

Station Three: Dessert and Coffee

Strawberry Shortcake

Color Palette and Decor

You guessed it—red, white, and blue. Plan to put a cluster of balloons on the mailbox or walkway of the hosting houses (and remember to leave lights on for approaching guests). Paper plates will make cleanup much easier; buy them in bulk and share with other hostesses. Use regular household items in unusual ways: Clean and recycle Campbell's soup cans to use as containers for plastic utensils; recycle diced-tomato cans and fill with fresh herbs for an inexpensive, but interesting, centerpiece. Then gather baby-food jars and, once scrubbed, use them as votive candle holders (labels can be left on or removed).

The Perfect Game or Activity

Between the moving, the eating, and the gift opening, this party is already packed with things to do. Take the pressure off setting up for baby shower games—just take the time to get acquainted or reacquainted with the neighbors.

Gifts That Work with This Theme

Get baby ready to explore the new neighborhood with these gift ideas:

- ✓ **Family Game Night.** Give a basket with an assortment of games and activities for families.
- ✓ **Tricycle.** This is for the day when baby is ready to explore the neighborhood.
- ✓ **Pack 'n Play.** Baby will be ready for an overnight stay with a trusted neighbor so Mom and Dad can have a date night.
- ✓ **Needs Calendar.** Create a calendar of the new mommy's needs—like carpooling duty, family meals, babysitting, and such. Have guests pitch in to help out by selecting a date and time to handle one or more of the posted needs.

Favors

Create a *Neighborhood Notebook* that contains pertinent information for the neighbors. It could include names of family members with birthdates, phone numbers, emergency numbers, babysitter information, even allergies. Save a page for favorite recommendations like best pizza parlor, best burgers, or where to get a good kid's haircut. Gather the information before the party—through phone calls or e-mails—then have it copied and spiral-bound at your local copy shop, and give one to each neighbor as they leave the party.

THEME IDEA 2 *The Red Wagon Food Challenge Shower*

Fans of the food television station will recognize the inspiration for this party idea. Stage your own cooking competition. In the original series, two chefs battle over a hot stove for a coveted title by cooking up a five-course meal that features a secret ingredient, such as shark or truffles. The challenge is that the ingredient must be used in every course, from appetizer to dessert. In this three-course version, the secret ingredient is, of course, baby food—from ground chicken to strained peas to soupy oatmeal.

Guests will be divided into teams and asked to create a menu and cook a meal from the grocery bag of ingredients they are handed—including jars of baby food. They will also be asked to create a babyish centerpiece for the serving table from a bag of craft supplies.

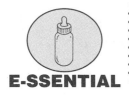

E-SSENTIAL

Don't forget to bring your video camera for the Whining Chef Food Challenge. You and the winning (or whining) team can star in your own version of a "foodie" TV episode. All the chefs, as well as the mom- and dad-to-be, will love watching reruns of this kitchen competition.

Setting It Up

Planning a culinary competition makes the cooking easier for the hostess, but requires some extra "prep" time in the area of organization. Make lists of the equipment you will need, such as three whisks, five spatulas, ten mixing bowls, as well as groceries, team members, and tasks. Set up stations around the party area for food preparation, cooking, supply storage, and busing. If you have only one stove (as most people do), create alternate cooking areas. Set up an outdoor grill, or use an electric frying pan on a protected table or counter with access to electricity. Create a station near your mixer and microwave oven. Press the toaster oven into service. Make sure that there are tools available at each location as well as hot mitts, dish towels, and a trash receptacle. When guests start cooking, you will be able to participate and enjoy both the process and the results.

The Red Wagon Food Challenge

Designate three judges for this competition.

Rules:

1. Hostess assembles a basic shopping list of ingredients for a three-course dinner (e.g., Mexican, Italian, French)—appetizer, entrée, and dessert.
2. Hostess provides beverages and secret ingredients—baby food, including jars of meats, vegetables, fruits, dry cereal, and fruit juice.
3. Hostess divides shopping list into groups of four or five items, which are purchased and brought by each guest.
4. At the start of the party, ingredients are placed on a kitchen table. Place the secret ingredients in a mini-red wagon (see Appendix A) covered with a cloth diaper.
5. Divide guests into two teams. Each team has ten minutes to develop a three-course menu based on the pool of ingredients on the table. No cookbooks are allowed!
6. When the timer goes off, have each team take turns selecting the ingredients they will need. Bartering and bargaining for desired ingredients are encouraged between teams.
7. Once the ingredients are dispersed, the secret ingredient is revealed. The secret ingredient must be used in every course.
8. Each team has one to one and a half hours to prepare and cook their meal. They will also have to create a centerpiece from the bag of baby items.
9. Each team must present their three dishes at the end of the cooking time. They will be rated on taste and presentation. Table décor and the centerpiece will also be judged.

Groceries and Ingredients

Determine the general theme concept that works best for your group, then make a list of the ingredients that will give the two teams a range of menu options for creating the three courses. For example: A Tex-Mex menu might include chips and salsa, tacquitos with guacamole and sour cream, fajitas and sizzling vegetables served with rice and beans, chicken mole with chili peppers, and banana flan for dessert. Here is a sample of some of the ingredients you might need for a themed dinner with a Tex-Mex flavor:

- ✓ **Beans and grains.** Black beans, pinto beans, rice
- ✓ **Produce.** Onions, fresh tomatoes, lettuce, corn, chili peppers, red and green bell peppers, jalapeño peppers, avocados, limes, lemons, bananas, shredded coconut
- ✓ **Canned goods.** Tomatoes, enchilada sauce, salsa, green chilis, olives
- ✓ **Seasonings.** Cilantro, chili powder, cumin, cinnamon, garlic, cayenne pepper, salt
- ✓ **Meat, poultry, and eggs.** Chicken, eggs, pork, ground beef, shrimp, or flank steak
- ✓ **Pantry items.** Masa harina (corn meal), flour, salt, pepper, sugar, vanilla, milk, oil, cooking spray, caramel sauce, cocoa powder, or chocolate sauce
- ✓ **Chips and wraps.** Blue or yellow corn tortilla chips and flour or corn tortilla flats in classic white, red tomato, or spinach flavors
- ✓ **Dairy products.** Sour cream, ice cream, whipped cream, shredded cheese, butter
- ✓ **Secret ingredients.** The five items of assorted baby foods, including jars of fruits, vegetables, and meats, as well as cereal, teething biscuits, and juices, will be given to each team; remember, they will be required to use all the secret ingredients.

Invitation Ideas and Script

Grab Your Spatulas and Recipes Too
We've Got a Little Competition for You!
Come to Celebrate Josh and Jen's
Best Recipe Yet—Baby Russell
Friday, February 16, 2008
At 6:00 in the evening
The Red Wagon Food Challenge will
Bestow the title of
The Whining Chef to the Winning Cook!
Please bring the following five ingredients

1. _____

2. _____

3. _____

4. _____

5. _____

R.S.V.P. to Kathy by February 1st.

Color Palette and Decor

Start with red and white, then you can adjust the color palette for this party as your chosen food theme dictates—add green if you are doing an Italian dinner or hot pink and orange if a fiesta is more to your liking. As the hostess, you may only need to provide a white table cloth (cloth, paper, or plastic); napkins (paper or cloth); and some red flatware, but you can influence the outcome of the centerpiece challenge by choosing colorful or color-coordinated items for the craft-supply bag.

The chefs and their teams will create the décor with the supplies you give them. For table décor, assemble a bag of supplies such as: rattles, ribbons, clothespins, disposable diapers, tape, scissors, tin foil, pipe cleaners, hot glue, paper clips, crepe, paper streamers, tissue paper, binkies, baby socks, or other baby items. Centerpieces can be "traditional"—a cluster of paper "flowers" crafted from tissue paper—or nontraditional—a baby carriage sculpted from tin foil and paper clips.

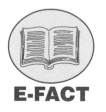

E-FACT

Don't forget to decorate with music. Add a layer of décor to your party's theme in the form of music. Have a techno-savvy guest prepare a CD of mixed songs that will add spice to the cooking, then keep them cranked up for the evening.

Gifts That Work with This Theme

Since the party focuses on food, focus the gift giving on feeding baby, too. Any of the following items will be great baby gifts:

- ✓ **Mini food processor.** Perfect for grinding up homemade yummies into baby-size bites
- ✓ **Baby-food-making kit.** Comes complete with chopping, blending, and heating devices as well as thermometer, freezing trays, an instruction guide, and baby food cook book
- ✓ **Feeding equipment.** Feeding bowl with matching cup, silver cup and spoon, bottle warmers, bottle brushes, or a breast pump
- ✓ **Baby equipment.** High chair, booster seat, breastfeeding support pillows (e.g., Boppie), burp cloths

Favors

Guests will love the opportunity to dress the part of the Whining Chef. Present everyone with a customized apron and hat before the competition heats up. You can stamp the hats with rubber stamps, have them silkscreened, or give people a set of markers and let them decorate their own. See *www.everydayeventplanner.com* for templates for chef's hats and aprons.

Have a trophy or trophies for the winning Whining Chef team. A wooden spoon (one for each team member) with the date and occasion printed on the handle is one idea. Another idea is to give out boxes of Hot Tamales (for a Tex-Mex finish) or Domori Italian chocolate bars.

THEME IDEA 3 | *The Red Wagon Community Diaper Drive*

For the mommy and baby-to-be who have everything they need, friends and family can still gather and give gifts. Try this celebratory shower with a strong social conscience—the community diaper drive. Instead of a traditional setting and décor, shower throwers will experience the joy of giving to those with greater need. This community shower is great for second- or third-time (or more) mothers. Diaper donations are encouraged; however, any baby item will be well-received and much-appreciated, from car seats to clothing, to cribs and bibs.

There are lots of bare bottoms without the bare necessities. Babies are born every day, in every community, whose parents cannot provide for all their basic needs. One of those needs is disposable diapers. These diapers are not a luxury for babies; they are a necessity. Infants use an average of twelve diapers per day (toddlers use about eight diapers per day), which translates to a cost of $100 per month for disposables. The Red Wagon Community Diaper Drive is a way to create an event that gives a hand to families in need. You can organize a diaper drive through your neighborhood, church, school, or service group.

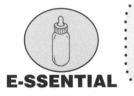

E-SSENTIAL

Typically, the drop-off sites are cardboard boxes or barrels located in school or church parking lots, community centers, or local businesses (e.g. coffee shops, grocery stores, etc.).

Setting It Up

The Red Wagon Diaper Drive can be set up in several ways, depending on the number of people you will have working on the project and the amount of time you wish to devote to collecting and delivering the diapers. The drive can be held on a single day (the shower day), or collection can take place over a period of time. In addition, you can have diapers dropped off at one location or several collection sites. You can stage the shower as the event that draws attention to the drive and raises awareness for the need for diapers. Start a diaper drive to coordinate with other community, school, or church events; for example, the school's Halloween Haunted House or Spring Carnival.

You will need to let the community know when the drive is taking place, who it will honor (the new baby's name goes here!) and the group that will benefit from it through posters, flyers, newsletters, the local newspaper, and even radio or television.

To set up the diaper-drive shower you will need to:

1. **Choose a charity.** Pick a group, organization, or agency who will be the recipient of the diapers you collect; this can be a charity the mom-to-be is involved in or a local charity in need. Ask if they have a

specific number of diapers they are in need of to help you determine what your event should aim for.

2. **Pick a date.** Plan for at least six to eight weeks lead time before the shower to organize and publicize the event. Coordinate the drive dates with the agency/group you have chosen.

3. **Determine a budget.** If you are planning to advertise, print flyers, order banners or balloons, or rent a delivery/collection truck you will need to figure out these costs first.

4. **Choose a drop-off or collection location(s).** Make arrangements for container placement, drop-off and pick-up.

5. **Create a publicity plan.** Make a list of area newspapers and local community groups that have bulletins (e.g. religious organizations, schools, chambers of commerce, etc.). Send a press release (via e-mail, snail mail, or fax) to town and regional papers and radio and television stations.

6. **Organize manpower.** You will need people to man the collection sites, pick-up donation bins or barrels, and hand out donation receipts. Create a volunteer list and calendar to keep scheduling on track.

7. **Keep communication lines open and accessible.** Create a master list of contact information and drive schedule to disperse to all volunteers. Include cell phone numbers for all volunteers. Verify dates and plan with collection sites and transportation teams. Have maps available for drivers with location(s) clearly marked.

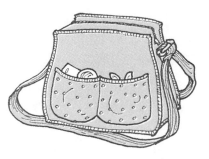

Invitation Idea and Script

Rather than a traditional invitation, this shower calls for a flyer. The Red Wagon Diaper-Drive Flyer should serve three purposes: 1. To inform the community about the date and time of the drive, as well as a contact person for more information; 2. To raise awareness about the need for diapers; and 3. To disclose the name of the group who will benefit from the donations. See *www.every dayeventplanner.com* for more ideas.

Color Palette and Décor

If your diaper drive will be held in a parking lot, balloons and banners are the best way to draw attention to the event. Clusters of balloons, either in baby pink and blue or a balloon arch will grab the eyes of passers by. Have a banner printed that says Diaper Drive and the name of the charity/organization you are collecting for. See *www.everydayeventplanner.com* for an example of a Diaper Drive banner.

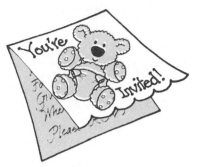

Chapter 16

Showers for Dads

TODAY'S DADS ARE not the figures of yesteryear, pacing in a hospital hallway, smoking cigarettes, and waiting to hear what kind of baby their wives have delivered. Modern dads are at the doctor visits, watching for the sonogram images, and at Mom's side, coaching her through contractions and back pain on the way to the delivery room. What's more, their roles as parents have also evolved. From crib construction to braided hair, these dads are involved in every aspect of child rearing. Here are some shower ideas that are strictly Y chromosome.

Who Can Use This Theme

The showers in this chapter are for dads—from the food (hearty, but simple), to the invitations (e-mails and text messages are fine), to the gift wrap (yes, you can give an unwrapped gift, just remove the price tag), to the locations, to the guest list (mostly men, although moms can be included, too). The logistical details focus on interesting activities rather than décor and fussy food presentation, and can be divided up among the guys; even a novice can get behind these showers. The testosterone-friendly ideas in this chapter will let new dads celebrate with their friends without swaths of pink and blue and those frilly shower games.

"Dads in the Digital Age" is a techie's dream party. Not only are the gift suggestions digital, but the activity—Geocaching, a GPS treasure hunt—makes the most of the techno-savvy roadsters. For the DIY (do-it-yourself) dad, an Extreme Nursery Makeover nails the fun together and yields a finished (or near-finished) baby's room. Finally, there's the Tailgate Shower, which teams up a ballgame, a parking lot, and a barbeque for the next generation of sports fans.

Regardless of their interests, these showers offer something for the spectrum of dads-to-be that will celebrate their new role.

Setting Up at Home

All three of these shower themes can be staged at a home. In the case of the digital shower, you could start and finish at home; however, there is a segment that involves a bit of travel. The nursery construction and décor shower must be done at the home of the new parents, while the sports-event shower just requires a wide-screen television and a remote control.

When setting up at home, décor is less important than clutter removal. Discard old mail, magazines, and newspapers, and put away clothes—even if they're tucked in a laundry basket in a closet.

Serving a meal at a man-shower can be as easy as fanning an assortment of take-out menus or as flavorful as fanning the barbeque flames. Forget your cholesterol concerns and go for the gusto of a real meal. If you have a good pizza parlor or burger joint in your neighborhood, you can order out. Set up stations for the bar and food presentation. A galvanized tub or your kitchen sink (clean, of course), filled with ice, can act as a beer and soft-drink station. Munchies and dips can go on the coffee table. Save a place for the main entree—whether it's pizza, a six-foot hero sandwich, or a platter of juicy steaks. Serve buffet style, every man for himself, but encourage offers of helping at cleanup time.

Setting Up Away from Home

Depending on your budget and circumstance, you can also take these showers out for a spin. Geocaching is done on the road, so you could pack lunches and snacks or arrange a pit stop at a favorite sports bar or hamburger stand. If the nursery work doesn't require major construction, you could assemble equipment or paint furniture at another location during the appointed shower time for later delivery to the baby's room.

The Tailgate Shower is a sports fan's dream. If you are a season-ticket holder, or even a one-game wonder, you can show your team spirit and say congratulations to a favorite buddy with this shower theme. Don't have a ticket? That's okay, too. You can set up your own sporting activity—play flag football, roller hockey, basketball, broom-ball (hockey played on ice with sneakers and brooms), Frisbee, golf, or beach volleyball—whatever game your group would enjoy.

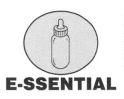

E-SSENTIAL

Some other ideas for sporting-event showers include a golf tournament, extreme Frisbee, rock-wall climbing, sky-diving, off-road biking, off-road ATVs, water polo, surfing, skiing, and camping.

Invitation Ideas

When inviting the guys to one of these man-friendly events, skip the formality of custom or preprinted invitations and get on the information highway. E-mails, phone calls, or text messages can convey all the necessary information in a flash and it won't get lost on a refrigerator or under a pile of bills or magazines. You should include the following information in any invitation:

- ✓ **Address.** Where the party will be held or where the group will meet.
- ✓ **Date and time.** List day of the week and date as well as the starting time and approximate ending time.
- ✓ **Timeline.** Let guests know when you will be leaving for a game, if you are expecting to return late, or have reservations at an eatery.
- ✓ **Costs.** Make guests aware of any expenses (dinner, rentals, tickets, etc.) or if they are expected to go in on a group gift.
- ✓ **Special equipment needed.** Tell your guests if they should bring hammers, a pound of nails, saws, paint brushes, a baseball glove, a GPS tracking system, or the like.
- ✓ **Contact information.** Let guests know how to respond that they are coming or not, and how they can reach you on the day of the shower. Remember, give multiple cell phone numbers, a home or work phone, or pager number, and be sure to include a way to handle emergency calls in case baby wants to arrive at party time.

THEME IDEA 1 · *Daddies in the Digital Age*

The advent of the Internet has allowed the scavenger hunt to go digital. Geocaching (pronounced geo-cashing) is a game that involves finding stashed treasures by using a global positioning system (GPS). This shower will take a bit of planning to set up, but will be well worth the effort for the digital adventurer.

Every cache location will have a log book to make entries regarding how the location was found or who found it; in fact, some caches consist of only a logbook. Some locations also have an online logbook to help track visitors and information. Cache items can include coins, jewelry, tickets, jokes, maps, CDs, pictures, tools, games, software, hardware, books, and so on. If you remove something from a cache, you must leave something in return.

There are two ways to set this up. The first is to join an online Web site (Geocache Clubs) and tap into existing locations of caches in your area. Download the "waypoints" (the exact latitudinal and longitudinal coordinates where the cache is located) that are near your party location. Make a list of the coordinates (there are downloadable software programs that make this easy) and give to the guests when they arrive. Unlike a road rally, guests will be following digital clues rather than road signs exclusively.

The other way to set up this shower is to use a company that specializes in team building through geocaching. These businesses set up the hunt, provide hand-held GPS systems with preprogrammed coordinates based on your group's interests, and handle all communication, log books and setup. See Appendix A for companies that offer this service.

Menu Ideas and Options

Since the travel element of this shower may place certain restrictions on the start time and the meal type and location, backpack snack packs for the car will provide the perfect solution. If you are inclined to bake, the cake-mix cookies have the "cache" of homemade and bake up in a jiffy. Add bottles of energy drinks and packages of sunflower seeds or corn nuts and your group is ready to hit the highway.

Daddies in the Digital Age Shower Menu

Hidden-Treasure Trek Mix
*Pretzels, Cheddar "Fish," Peanuts, Popcorn, and Cereal Flavored
with Grill Seasonings and Worcestershire Sauce*

Energy Drinks
such as Red Bull, Vitamin Water, Gatorade, or Iced Coffee

Setting It Up

There's not much need for centerpieces and streamers at this shower, but there is a definite need for communication between the guests. Provide each guest or vehicle with a packet of information that includes cache waypoints, cell phone numbers, and general rules for the game. Also give names and addresses of rest stops and restaurants in case anyone strays from the group.

Since many caches are themed, plan on leaving something behind that suits the theme. For example: If you have chosen a cache that has coins, you should plan to leave another coin in its place.

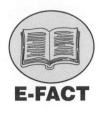

GPS systems are available at boat supply stores, camping supply stores, on the Web, and even at Amazon.com. Some phones even come with GPS systems in them. There are a number of books that cover picking a GPS system for outdoor activities.

The Perfect Game or Activity

A Geocaching Digital-Game Competition is the activity designed for this party. The main activity coordinator will let guests know what maps and supplies are needed and will assign groups to the cars or trucks that will be used—everyone should have a buddy with them. Your geocaching day will include some kind of meal and may also include some gift giving, so take these shower elements into account when setting up a time to start and end this shower.

When choosing which caches to hunt for, consider their size and location. This information is included on the online postings, which also list the degree of difficulty of the surrounding terrain and other pertinent information. If the location is off the beaten path and will require a bit of a hike, you should figure this into the timeline. Take into account the travel time between cache sites and the number of sites you plan to visit in a few hours.

Geocaching has four main components: choosing the cache location, planning the trip, going on the hunt, and reporting the find.

✓ **Choose the location.** This phase is done on the Internet. Since many caches are hidden away from the road, locating them will take some work. Research information about the cache includes online notes from other geocachers about what they encountered to find a particular location.

✓ **Plan the trip.** Your GPS system is only one of the tools you will need to find treasure. Road and topographical maps are recommended, especially if the site is off-trail. Most systems have a compass, but an old-fashioned one should be part of your equipment kit. Be prepared for climate changes, bathroom breaks, and carry snacks and water.

- ✓ **Go on the hunt.** Most navigational systems will easily get you within a mile or less of the treasure spot; however, the last part of the trek can be the most challenging. Geocachers agree that the last one hundred feet are the hardest. Make sure to mark your vehicle position in your GPS device to make the return to the car faster and easier.
- ✓ **Report the find.** After noting your discovery in the logbook at the site, you may choose to take something from the cache. The rule here is: If you take something you must leave something. Return the storage container to its original position and cover it so that it is as you found it. Use your digital camera to take a picture of the site or anything unusual or interesting that you encounter on the way. When you return home, you will make an entry online or e-mail the cache originator.

This relatively new adventure activity can be tailored to the needs and interests of any group. And who knows, this may become a new hobby for the group—you might even decide to start a club!

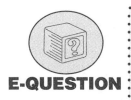

E-QUESTION

Can I hide my own cache?
Yes, you can. Geocaching is a global phenomenon, and there are locations all over the world, each one set up by ordinary folks. Every site should have a log book and be protected from the elements. See geocaching Web sites for the best way to set up your own cache.

Gifts That Work with This Theme

There are a gaggle of digital gifts for baby on the market today. Baby monitors, DVD players with Baby Einstein programs, even digital thermometers are widely available. Other ideas include:

- ✓ **Nursery monitor.** Comes with audio and video feeds. Some systems allow offsite monitoring through a secure Web site.
- ✓ **DVD player.** The new baby may be too young for Baby Einstein, but the new dad can catch up on the latest DVD until baby is ready to dictate what to play.

✓ **Camping gear.** Get baby ready for a trek or outdoor adventure with a backpack baby carrier, car shade, and thermal blankets.

Favors

The guys may not expect a party favor, but surprise them with customized mouse pads featuring the party theme or funny photos of the group. You can also give custom keychains, baseball hats, or notebooks. See Appendix A for resources.

THEME IDEA 2 | *Extreme Nursery Makeover*

Okay, guys—grab your tool belt, hammer, and level; baby's getting a new nursery! A little coordination, some paint chips, an Allen wrench, a crate of unassembled furniture, and a group of construction-savvy friends are all you will need to build this shower. To pull off a productive working shower, you will need to systematize some details in advance.

Menu Ideas and Options

There are two options for preparing a meal for the makeover workers: eat in or order out. If you have a large crew, and you plan to order something, be sure to call in an order well in advance and order generously—hammering makes you hungry. Cooking at home is an option if the project won't interfere with your kitchen. Try this sandwich favorite to satisfy even the hungriest of guests.

Extreme Nursery Makeover Shower Menu

Classic Reuben Sandwich
Corned Beef, Sauerkraut, Swiss Cheese, and Russian Dressing on Rye Bread

Macaroni Salad
Elbow Pasta with Pimiento, Olives, Chopped Egg, and Celery

Cake-Mix Cookies

Setting It Up

As the carpenters say, "Measure twice, cut once." Planning is everything with this project party. Experts recommend setting up work areas for different jobs. Each area should have a work surface (table, saw horses, etc.), access to electricity if needed, good light, materials and supplies, and a trash container. Keep dust-producing jobs like sawing and sanding away from paint and finish areas.

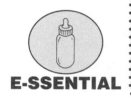

E-SSENTIAL

Lots of folks don't feel comfortable with a hammer, but they know how to wield a broom. Invite them to come for the meal and assign these "angels" the task of cleanup. By the end of the workday, their fresh energy and unique skills will be a much-appreciated contribution to the project.

Here are some issues to consider when setting up a makeover project party:

✓ **Size and scope.** Does the room require cosmetic or construction work? Determine the scale of the project.

✓ **Coordinate with Mom.** Find out mommy's choices for colors, décor style, furniture and fixture placement, and so on before you start any part of the project. Get samples and her approval first. You can surprise her with a job well done, but not with an unplanned nursery.

✓ **Create a project timeline.** Figure out all the jobs that need to be tackled, spackled, and built. Estimate the number of hours needed to complete the tasks chosen for the workday (and be realistic!) and the manpower needed to complete them. List projects in the order they should be done. Pair up talent with tasks—put your friend the cabinet maker on woodwork, not drywall.

✓ **Create a supply list.** Workers can't work without the proper tools and supplies. Appoint a "foreman" to oversee work, keep supplies coming, and assist where needed.

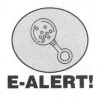

Remember to have extra extension cords, duct tape, trash bags, brooms, dustpans, work lights for dark spaces like closets, plastic or cloth covers to protect baby's things from dust and grime, and have a hose handy (to rinse things off at the end of the day).

✓ **Safety first.** Have a safety plan and a well-stocked first-aid kit on site.

✓ **Post a schedule.** Put up a schedule on the "worksite" and, if possible, send it with the invitation. Include jobs, workers, timeline, and any tools or supplies needed.

✓ **Feed the group.** An army moves on its stomach and so will this make-over team. Plan to have coffee and bagels, water and soft drinks, sandwiches, snacks, and whatever else will safely satisfy hunger and thirst. A well-fed team is a productive team.

✓ **Start with deconstruction.** Empty the room of boxes and beds, tear out the carpet, and do any demolition first.

✓ **Clean up between phases.** Keeping dust and dirt to a minimum will make the environment easier to work in.

✓ **Keep Mom out.** Many paints and glues have noxious properties that shouldn't be inhaled, especially by pregnant women. Provide masks for workers to protect them against fumes and dust, if necessary.

✓ **Give everyone a job.** Standing around idly is frustrating, so have jobs planned for all skill levels of the guests/friends in attendance. Recycled furniture can be painted, polished, and refurbished. New furniture and equipment, from changing tables to strollers, may need assembly. Drawers can be lined with shelf paper, and decorative knobs and pulls can replace tired, worn ones. Pictures and curtains can be hung. Make the most of any helping hands available.

✓ **Keep the energy up with music.** Whether you listen to jazz or rap, on an iPod or a boom box, keep things moving with music. If music is not your style, turn on the ballgame.

✓ **Celebrate at the end.** Take a picture of the work crew to add to baby's book. This labor of love and friendship will be long remembered and well used.

Gifts That Work with This Theme

Guests have already given the most precious gift, the gift of time; however, if they wish to present the parents-to-be with something more, nursery items are the choice du jour for this shower. Many home-furnishing and baby stores have gift registries that include nursery-décor items. Consider pitching in for a rocking chair, bookshelf, or even a crib to complete the room.

- ✓ **Curtains, bumpers, and pillows.** Store-bought or hand-made curtains, along with coordinating crib bumpers, sheets, and the like, will add the finishing touches to baby's room.
- ✓ **Area rug.** A great gift for a room with hardwood floors or as an additional layer of interest over wall-to-wall carpeting.
- ✓ **Specialty furniture.** Swivel gliders, traditional rockers, and toy chests will be used and appreciated by parents and baby alike.

Favors

What would be more needed after a day of reaching, bending, and hauling than a goodies bag of home remedies for life's aches and pains! Fill an empty one-gallon paint can with these items to send home with the guys:

- ✓ Band Aids
- ✓ Tube of pain-relief cream
- ✓ Cold/hot compress
- ✓ Beer and corn nuts

THEME IDEA 3 **_Tailgate Shower_**

Tailgating is an art form, just ask any sports fan. Take the new dad or dad-to-be to a game and shower him with a tailgating party. Whether your team is nationally recognized or locally loved, a college alma mater or opening day on the high school football field, you can show the father-to-be how to party like a pro. This is more than just a few sandwiches in a cooler—this is a no-holds-barred grilling and eating extravaganza and then a ball game!

If the idea of a tailgating shower appeals to your sports-minded spirit, but you don't have tickets to a stadium sport, stage your own game. Get friends together for a friendly afternoon of baseball that starts with a tailgate party and ends with a game. So pack up the grill, load up the SUV, and head for the ball park.

Menu Ideas and Options

If grilling is your style, consider these menu ideas that will definitely impress the guys.

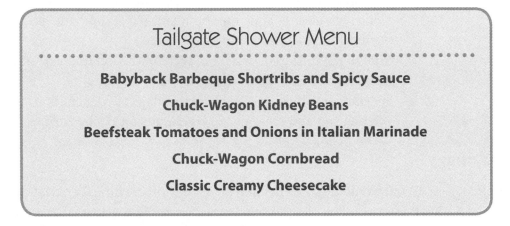

Tailgate Shower Menu

Babyback Barbeque Shortribs and Spicy Sauce

Chuck-Wagon Kidney Beans

Beefsteak Tomatoes and Onions in Italian Marinade

Chuck-Wagon Cornbread

Classic Creamy Cheesecake

Setting It Up

Tailgaters are serious fans—about their team and about their food. This is no time for planning on the fly; stocking up takes time and organization. Most tailgaters arrive at the ballpark three to four hours early and stay for an hour or two after the game. Including game time, this event will cover an entire day and range of meals.

✓ **Plan menus and supply lists ahead.** You will need food supplies, cooking equipment, and safe storage (sealed containers with lots of ice) for two to three meals. Make sure you prepare not only a grocery list but also a list of cooking essentials. Check off supplies as you load them into your vehicle. Assign items and groceries to other partygoers.

✓ **Prepare food items the night before.** Some foods may require marinating, chopping, tenderizing, or baking ahead of time. Get everything ready and packed in disposable containers (except for perishables) the evening before the game.

✓ **Set the schedule for cooking and eating.** Allow about one hour to set up grills and food-preparation areas. Food should be ready to eat about ninety minutes before the game starts. This will give everyone a chance to eat, clean up, and cool down the grill. Once the game is over, make sure your parking spot is spotless.

✓ **Get there early.** Tailgating is not for the lazy or faint-of-heart. Get to the parking lot early to pick a prime spot (near grass or at the end of a row), get set up, and get cooking—especially if you are roasting a three-hour brisket!

✓ **Decorate the space.** You are celebrating a friend and his team. Fly a flag so partygoers can find you in a sea of cars. Throw a team-logo'd tablecloth or blanket over the food table. Paper plates and napkins are available with lots of team insignias; pick up a package of napkins, matching plates and cups, and coordinating cutlery.

✓ **Dress like a team.** Ask guests to show their true "colors" by wearing team gear, from jerseys to hats.

Gear You Will Need

If you've tailgated before, you may already have a well-stocked garage. If you are a tailgating novice, you can find lots of gear at your local camping store. The difference between tailgate cooking and campsite cooking is scale and equipment. Die-hard tailgaters have some serious equipment—fryers, supergrills, hammocks, tables, lounge chairs, even hot tubs. Check out this list of basic gear:

✓ **Propane grill.** This is easier to cool down and eliminates the need to dispose of hot coals that can take days to fully cool.

✓ **Cooler.** A must-have for tailgating. Stores meat and food perishables. Keeps beverages cool. Most tailgaters will need more than one.

✓ **Serving and seating.** You will need a place to do some food preparation, serve the food, and sit down to eat.

✓ **Weather guards.** Rain, sleet, snow, and heat are all potential factors in your tailgating enjoyment. Canopies (for sun and rain), umbrellas, rain gear, sun block, and blankets should have a place on your basic supply list.

✓ **In case of emergency.** First-aid kit, jumper cables, toilet paper, antacid (nothing's worse than a stomach full of barbeque and a long ride home!), a small generator, flashlight, and fully charged cell phone.

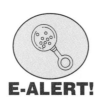

E-ALERT!

Never, never, never serve any food on a platter that has held raw meat until it has been thoroughly washed with hot, soapy water. Raw meat marinades should not be used as "gravy." If you wish to serve the marinade, bring it to a boil and serve hot over the cooked food. Food handlers should wash hands after touching raw meat, but before touching any other food or serving pieces.

Gifts That Work with This Theme

Initiate the new baby into his or her proud papa's sports interest with baby team gear and equipment.

✓ **Baby mitts.** The adorable baseball mitts come in brown (original), pink, and blue.

✓ **Team blanket.** Have the family name (or baby's name, if it's been decided) embroidered onto a fleecy team-style blanket.

✓ **Game cards.** Sports-card manufacturers produce card sets each year. Give a complete set and watch who becomes famous and who bites the dust!

✓ **Collegiate gear.** Bedeck baby in mom or dad's alma mater layette wear.

Favors

If you are inclined to give the assembled guests a remembrance of the day, consider thermal drink sleeves in your team's colors—you may even find them with the team's logo on them. For the avid tailgater crowd, a special meat rub or barbeque sauce will also be a hit.

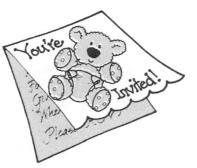

Chapter 17

Showers for Urban Über-Babes

SOMETIMES A GIRL, especially a pregnant one, just wants to have fun. These sexy-in-the-city celebrations are certainly for the mom-to-be, but instead of focusing strictly on baby, they turn a flirty false eyelash to the gal doing all the work. Grab a lipstick and stilettos for these sophisticated and über-chic urban showers.

Who Can Use This Theme

While these showers were conceived with a big city vibe, they can be modified to suit any urban or suburban setting. The concept here is to have a day with the girls—no husbands or boyfriends, no kids or carpools to worry about. Plan these showers earlier rather than later in the pregnancy as shopping, touring, and gallery hopping can be too strenuous in the last trimester. Baby will not be forgotten, but this is about the Maternity Girl.

The first shower, Phat and Phabulous: The Maternity Girl's a Fashionista, applauds the ever-expanding waistline and enhances mama's wardrobe at the same time. Girlfriends gather with a dual purpose—shop before the baby drops and accessorize the mama! This event can be staged in a trendy city shopping district, favorite department store, or your local mall.

Next is the Maternity Girl Goes "Tourista" Shower—where the mama and her friends take on the role of tourists for a few hours. This shower can range from a historical tour of interesting architectural buildings to a culinary walking tour of a specific city district to see the sights and sample the flavors to a private tour of a museum collection. Plan a movable feast by scheduling stops at street vendors or off-beat eateries along the way.

Finally, there's the Maternity Girl's Guide to Urban Artistas—a party that gives birth to creativity, crafts, or jewelry. From gallery hopping to art or craft classes, this shower is about expressing your inner artist. Artist colonies have sprung up all over the country, so this shower doesn't have to stay within the city limits.

Setting Up at Home

Most city dwellers will laugh at the idea of having a large group of people in their home. Urban living tends to create small living space. If you live in a studio apartment, tenth-floor walk-up, or tiny loft, don't panic; take this shower downtown (or uptown as the case may be).

You can set up the accessory party in your living room, kitchen, or bedroom, even if they are all the same room—all you will need is access to a mirror and a pitcher of mocktails (pink-grapefruit flirtinis, of course). The Artistas' Shower can also be held at home, as long as you have a simple project and enough room for each guest to have a lap-sized workspace.

What's in a pink–grapefruit flirtini?
This is an easy, breezy mocktail that's as refreshing as it is pretty. Take one part pink-grapefruit juice, one part cranberry juice, and a squeeze of lime and shake well. Serve in a sugar-rimmed martini glass with a whole cranberry and a thin slice of lime for garnish.

Setting Up Away from Home

The great advantage to living in a city is that the city is your living space. The little boutique around the corner can play hosting venue to dress your friend. Take her shopping in a trendy district, set her up in a dressing room, and let friends bring the outfits to her. Recharge after shopping at a nearby café—remember to make reservations if your group is a crowd or the café is a crowd favorite. For the art-loving mama, a shower that includes either viewing art or a hands-on class may be right up her gallery. Galleries offer both prescheduled and private showings, which are often guided by art aficionados who can provide colorful history, insights, and commentary about the pieces on display.

Invitation Ideas and Script

Celebrate the Maternity Girl in high style with a high-fashion invitation. Try paper-doll invitations that can be printed on cardstock, cut out, and dolled up to suit any style.

Lauren's a Maternity Girl!
Come help us celebrate her journey to
Phat and Phabulous
Friday, January 30th

For THEME 1 add: We're getting this Mama all dolled up! The day will include shopping, nibbling, gossiping, and accessorizing—Dress appropriately but Phabulously!

Or for THEME 2 add: We're taking mama on a walking tour (or culinary tour, bus tour, etc.), so grab your camera and come play "tourista" with us.

Or for THEME 3 add: It's an afternoon of creativity with a colorful palette and palette-pleasing delights—bring an art smock and make something Phabulous!

Since these showers are on the move rather than stationary, your invitations *are* the décor. They will set the fashion pace for the rest of the party. You can tweak the paper-doll invitation design depending on the theme idea you choose. Consider fashion icon paper-dolls, like Grace Kelly, Jacqueline Kennedy, Princess Diana, or Carrie Bradshaw for the shopping-day invitation (See Appendix A). If you are taking a historical architecture tour, use paper dolls representing fashions from the same era as the buildings you will be touring.

THEME IDEA 1 | *Phat and Phabulous: The Maternity Girl's a Fashionista*

The concept behind this shower is to give the mama-to-be a day to develop or expand her personal style and maybe her maternity attire, too. Let the best friends be the stylists as the group conquers fashion fearlessly. This shower can be planned earlier in the pregnancy to give her a chance to prepare a fashion-forward work (or play) wardrobe.

If you are in close proximity to an urban hub, you can plan a day trip to the city. If you're a city dweller, plan to stop and shop at nearby boutiques. A variation on this theme is to invite guests to share their gently used maternity clothes.

Menu Ideas and Options

You are going to be out and about in the city, so take a Zagat's guide with you and find a trendy café or landmark eatery, or ask locals for the name of a favorite hot spot. For hard-core shoppers, leaving the store is not an option, so hit the store cafeteria; but don't be surprised if your favorite department store's fuel stop becomes your favorite restaurant—there has been a retro resurgence of the lunch counter in many high-end department stores. Many department stores have given over their cafés to high-end chefs who bring new flavors to the old lunchroom. Dishes from designer sandwiches to decadent chocolate dessert bars grace the updated menus.

The Perfect Game or Activity

Shopping with girlfriends for a maternity "layette" needs a plan—no unfocused meandering through sale racks. The mama-to-be needs to get in, get out, and get what she needs to look "phantastic" for the rest of the pregnancy.

Maternity clothes are designed to fit the ever-expanding waistline, but over the course of nine months, the pregnant woman will need clothes for each stage as well as seasonal pieces and perhaps a special occasion or career outfit or two. The categories that should be considered are: underwear, sleepwear, casual wear, career wear, outerwear, dress-up, accessories, and shoes.

The Maternity Girl's "Layette":

✓ **Underwear.** Mama will need underwear for each trimester. During the first trimester, she can probably wear regular bikinis and hiphuggers, but in the second trimester, she may want to splurge on a few new pairs. By the third trimester, good-old-fashioned granny pants may be the order of the day, especially if she likes her undies to cover the bump. Bras are a must, even if she doesn't normally wear one. She will probably need to have two or three for the first half of the pregnancy and may need a larger size during the last three months.

✓ **Sleepwear.** Some women feel sexy during pregnancy and others do not. Consider having some fun lingerie as well as a couple of loose-fitting cotton nightshirts. Depending on the season, a bathrobe or sweats may also be necessary.

✓ **Casual wear.** This category will make up an important component of the pregnancy wardrobe. There are many choices in all ranges of styles and price points now available. During the first trimester, pants or skirts that sit at the natural waistline may still fit if the waist is left unbuttoned. By the fifth month, Mama will need either low-rise or bell-banded pants and skirts. Two pairs of jeans and some soft cotton pants—either sweats, yoga pants, or leggings—will be much used throughout the pregnancy. Casual tops can be specific to maternity wear or simply larger sizes of a favorite brand or style of T-shirt, sweatshirt, or hoodie. Splurge on a good-fitting pair of jeans that can do double duty when mixed with a career jacket and top.

✓ **Career wear.** This is another component of the maternity wardrobe that will need attention. Help Mom evaluate her business-outfit needs carefully. Second- and third-trimester dressing will require three bottoms—two pants and a skirt, and five to seven tops—including a jacket or two, if the weather will warrant it. Plan to layer, as ever-changing hormone levels can cause sweats and chills.

✓ **Outerwear.** Depending on the region she lives in, Mama will need at least one or two seasonal jackets or coats. Consider a flattering style that is somewhat loose-fitting and is not strictly maternity—since most good coats can last for more than one season.

✓ **Dress-up.** It is probably unlikely that a fashionista Mama will go nine whole months without a wedding or other social occasion that requires a fancy dress. Today's Maternity Girl can look superchic in one of the many styles and fabrics now in vogue.

✓ **Accessories.** This is the good stuff in the one-size-fits-all department. Consider scale when choosing accessories because mama's body will have a new shape. Big earrings, chunky necklaces, elegant scarves, and bold bracelets all scream fashion and take the focus off the waistline.

✓ **Shoes.** Start with comfort. During pregnancy, the same hormones that get the pelvis ready to deliver that bundle of joy also cause the joints in the feet to expand, sometimes as much as a size. The ever-widening girth also can make Mama off balance. Lower heels, cushiony soles, and wider widths will be needed throughout the pregnancy.

Shopping Strategy:

✓ **Make a list.** Create a list of needs, wants, and sizes.
✓ **What does she need?** Next figure out what the maternity girl could use to complete her layette, and what her budget will allow.

✓ **What can she borrow?** Ask friends, sisters, cousins, and coworkers to share a gently used outfit. You can even make this request on the invitation and ask them to bring dry-cleaned items to the party.

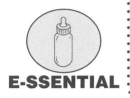

E-SSENTIAL

Show the belly! Maternity girls today are not afraid to show their shape. When dressing the bump, don't go too baggy; it ends up looking sloppy and adds bulk. Buy the size she needs for fit—forget the size numbers. One-color dressing creates a more slimming line and makes for easy mixing, matching, and accessorizing.

Gifts That Work with This Theme

Gifts for this shower can be for the baby, but the focus is on the mom, so give fashion a chance. Boost her self-confidence and fashion flair with any one of these gift ideas.

✓ **Jewelry.** Funky bracelets, fabulous earrings, interesting pins and brooches.

✓ **Handbags.** Sometimes a bag in an off-beat color or shape can make an outfit. Some of the new diaper bags are cuter than the handbags, so look into this option.

✓ **Scarves or hats.** For sun or sleet, these accessories are necessary and fashionable.

THEME IDEA 2 | *Maternity Girl Goes Tourista*

One of the great advantages of living in a cosmopolitan area is the wealth of sites, sounds, and flavors waiting to be discovered. This shower concept is simple: Gather friends to take a first look or a closer look at the attractions that make a city unique.

The tour could be a free-ranging exploration of the many forms of architecture in a neighborhood or a walking tour of historic places (e.g., the Freedom Trail in Boston, or Cannery Row in Monterey).

A culinary city walk is a delicious and informative way to tour the town. In New York, you can tour the meatpacking district and see where the Oreo cookie was invented. In San Francisco, you can take a cable car to the Buena Vista Café where Irish Coffee was invented, then head to Ghirardelli Square for an outrageous hot-fudge sundae. All along the way, aromas and food samplings are available. Meals and tastings are included in the price of guided tours, or do a little neighborhood research and map out your own.

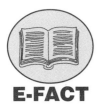

E-FACT

Tour companies can be an excellent resource for city tours and culinary adventures. You can find companies that will offer basic information and a map, prepackaged and available for everyone on the tour, or you can schedule a private-party tour complete with a knowledgeable guide. Some tour companies will even pack a snack for a price.

For the high-brow set, a museum tour is a perfect solution. From the Met to MOMA, Mama will love one last free-wheeling jaunt through valuables and breakables without fear of tiny, grasping hands leaving sticky handprints on priceless artifacts. Pick up bags of hot peanuts at a street vendor for a snack and make reservations for lunch at a nearby café. Many museums have eateries on premise; check out their menus online before you embark on your journey.

The Perfect Games or Activity

When planning this shower, a few elements will need consideration to make it a pleasant experience for everyone, especially the mom.

✓ **Select considerately.** History buffs may love a museum, foodies will love a culinary tour, but not all Mom's friends will have the same tastes and interests as the rest of the group. Get consensus from the group before you make firm plans and reservations.

✓ **Mode of travel.** Walking tours are nice in good weather but could be impossible if it's horribly hot, cold, or wet. Many cities have sightseeing buses that give touristas a comfortable perch from which to enjoy the sites. Some cities have amphibious vehicles that show you the sites by land and sea—check out Boston's Duck Tours.

✓ **Length of tour.** Determine how long the tour will take. Walking for two hours with baby on board may not be the mama's cup o' tea. Find out if mobile tours allow you to get on and off during the trip.

✓ **Plan for breaks.** Stretching crampy legs and bathroom breaks are a must for pregnant gal-pals. Make sure the restroom stops are adequate and acceptable.

✓ **Dress appropriately.** Plan for weather changes and bring sunscreen if you will be outside for any length of time.

Check out tour ideas at your local bookstore, chamber of commerce, visitor's bureau, or library. Many Web sites also provide information about upcoming tours, exhibits, and other attractions.

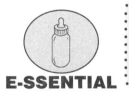

E-SSENTIAL

When exploring a big city from a culinary point of view, plan to do a little research before you take that first bite. Knowing the district's food history, the chef's food philosophy, and local legends and myths related to stops along the way will turn a walk into an adventure.

Gifts That Work with This Theme

Get the new mama some of the items she will need to pack as she embarks on her maternity journey.

✓ **Hospital bag.** An attractive bag filled with delivery-room needs like lollipops, massage oil, and socks.

✓ **Overnight bag.** Encourage future travel for Mom and Dad with a new overnight bag.

✓ **A taste of the tour.** Give a gift that reminds Mama of her day with friends—Seattle's Best coffee, a Napa wine, or Santa Barbara's olive oil, to name a few.

Favors

Remind friends of your day spent together every time they travel with a custom luggage tag. Order them personalized or make your own with the art from the invitation.

See *www.everydayeventplanner.com* for luggage tag designs.

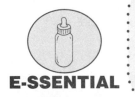

E-SSENTIAL

If taking in an entire tour is too much, try seeing just one site. Choose a one-stop favorite location to visit or revisit. Ride a cable car, take a ferry, stop at a mission or historical landmark, then head for lunch or dinner!

THEME IDEA 3 | *The Maternity Girl's Guide to Urban Artistas*

This shower is the art of the party. Create an occasion that inspires creativity with bracelet-making by day and gallery-hopping by night.

Art galleries present interesting and eclectic collections of local, national, and international art, which can range from paintings to sculptures to jewelry to woodworking and ceramics. Many locales with a preponderance of galleries coordinate gallery-hopping events one night a week. Guests can take a glass of wine or Perrier and meander through the exhibits.

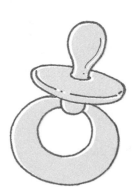

If your area has an active artist colony or society, you can visit the creative stomping grounds during an Open Studios Tour. These events give the public a chance to see the art being created and even to purchase a piece or two.

As an alternative to the gallery-hopping shower, you can stage your own open studio or take an art class through a college, recreation department, or retail store. A project that is exciting and easy, regardless of the guests' skill levels, is bracelet-making. In a few hours, friends will leave with wearable art.

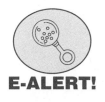

E-ALERT!

Art projects can be a joy if you are confidant and inspired artistically, but they are daunting and intimidating to those among us who prefer other creative outlets. When choosing a project for a group, bring pictures and ideas that the creatively challenged can copy or imitate. It will take the fear out of the process and let the fun in.

The Perfect Game or Activity

There are many options to choose from when selecting the type of art project or class you want to stage. Check out course catalogs and local newspapers for information about upcoming classes. The ceramics lounge can now be found in cities large and small. A reservation, some wine and cheese, and a bottle of sparkling blackberry soda are all you need to spell success. Each person can make something for Mom or baby or can keep the finished work for themselves and bring a gift instead.

Jewelry-making supplies and tools can be found at craft stores, and this activity is a terrific way to spend an afternoon with friends. One project that can be handled at any skill level is putting together a Slinky-style bracelet—the kind that involve stringing beads onto a multicoiled wire that looks like the original Slinky. Directions for these bracelets are available where you purchase the supplies. There are also jewelry project kits available.

How to Set Up a Bracelet-Making Party

1. **Setup stations.** Each guest will need a flat surface as big as a TV tray to set up their work station. Each station should have a piece of light-colored felt (8" × 10") to work on, which keeps the beads from rolling off the table.

2. **Have the right tools and supplies.** Jewelry supply and craft stores sell specific pliers for twisting and clamping wires. Have one set of tools (consisting of long-nose pliers, a wire cutter, and a crimper) for every four people. You will also need 22-gauge coiled memory wire for bracelets. Each bracelet will need about 20 inches, which is about five coils. Multiply this times the number of guests.

3. **Shop for beads and baubles.** Beads come in vials or in larger bags. Each bracelet will need at least a vial's worth of beads to complete. You should plan on having at lest ten colors of 2mm beads (glass is prettier than plastic, but it is more expensive), and five to seven signature baubles per bracelet. Also get metal charms, initials, symbols, or sparkles to add personality to these creations. Put beads and baubles in a clean muffin tin or ice-cube tray to sort, separate, and disperse to the group.

4. **Precut bracelet wire.** Allow seven to ten loops for each bracelet. Have them cut before the guests arrive.

5. **Embrace all designs.** There is no wrong way to make these fun and funky embellishments. Beads can be placed with precision and pattern or at random—both will produce a beautiful result.

Gifts That Work with This Theme

For this shower, have each guest bring a silver charm for a bracelet for the mom. It could be a girlfriend memory, a baby-related icon, or an engraved disk with a date, saying, or baby's name. Have each friend present the charm to Mom and explain the story behind it. Attach charms yourself or arrange to have a jeweler do it.

Another great gift idea is a wall-mounted frame that actually opens like a cabinet—making storing and changing pictures a snap.

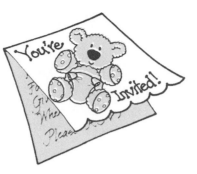

Chapter 18

e-Showers: From Virtual to Desktop to "Lap-Top"

TRANSPORTATION AND INTERNET commerce have expanded the way showers can be planned, attended, and even hosted. Pregnancy is no longer a sentence to stay home and get ready for baby to arrive, so moms-to-be are working right up to the first contraction. And since babies can come at any time, sometimes there's no time for a shower. "Lap-top" showers, when baby attends on mama's lap, can be a great solution for the babies who can't wait to get here. The showers in this chapter have been designed to take hostesses from virtual to desktop to "lap-top" without a single labor pain.

Who Can Use This Theme

Anyone with access to the Internet, television, or a BlackBerry can manage the details of these events. The Virtually Virtual Shower allows a "remote" hostess to activate a plan and send a finished party anywhere in the world with a post office or FedEx delivery. Coffee-Break Contractions is designed for the working girl and her pod-mates. Sure, its only fifteen minutes long, but it can be her fifteen minutes of fame in the workplace. And don't forget, there's the party you can't plan for in advance, the "Lap-top" shower. There are many cultures that don't shower mother and baby until after the birth, but this is really more of a visit with presents than a classic baby shower. There are some rules of etiquette for visits after the birth and some real-time, roll-up-your-sleeves ideas to help Mom deal with the reality of bringing baby home.

THEME IDEA 1 | *The Virtually Virtual Shower*

Plan a shower that you won't attend but will attend to—a virtual shower. Thanks to the Internet, you can locate almost any kind of dinner and send it anyplace where mail delivery trucks trek. This is a lucky break for the hostess with the most-est who's two states away, since it means that you can send the new parents-to-be a gift certificate to their favorite bistro or send them an order of their favorite ribs to enjoy right at home. And while they're licking barbeque sauce off their fingers, moms-to-be can open the lovely baby blanket you had sent from the gift registry so that it arrives at the same time. A gift, a meal, and a baby-on-the-way—it's a shower; if you can think it virtually, you can make it a reality.

As the virtual hostess, you won't be there to control the details, so don't try. Keep things limited to a few elements, and then bask in the knowledge that you have given a mom-to-be a shower she'll be talking about for years. This is the ultimate online experience for baby showers and the major planning is just a few clicks away.

In addition to being a virtual hostess, you may want to consider hosting a Web page for the parents-to-be. For the digitally minded, it may only take an hour to set up, but it could include photos of mom-and-dad-to-be, other siblings, pregnancy updates, baby-item wish lists, shower information, potential baby names, and even a baby blog. Send out an e-mail blast to family and friends announcing the birth of the Web page and any security information they will need to access it.

Setting It Up

The key elements for the virtual hostess to plan are the food and the gift; then you can add on flowers, favors, and fun. There are a number of ways to make this work:

✓ **You pay; they plan.** In this scenario, you do a little research, either on the Internet or by placing a well-timed call to the dad-to-be to find out the mom's personal preferences or local favorites. Then you call or e-mail to have a gift certificate sent to the happy parents, who pick their best night to go out to dinner. You send a baby gift from their online registry, and you're done. Depending on your budget, you can increase the amount of the gift certificate so they can bring friends or family. This works well for the mom who has a busy work or social schedule.

✓ **You pay; you plan; you send her out for a party.** This approach involves you setting everything up for a party at a location that is not in a home. You could arrange for a dinner with friends on a specific evening or a supper followed by a concert. Contact the expectant mother or father to get some preliminary particulars such as date availability, general mobility, and her approval for the event details before you punch in a credit card number and hit send.

✓ **You pay; you plan; you send it to her at home.** The doorbell rings, and the party arrives. Whether it's a shower for the girls, a backyard barbeque for family, or breakfast in bed, this party comes to her. Since you aren't limited by restaurant guidelines and restrictions, you can send as much in the way of details as suits your virtual fantasy. Flowers, plates with matching napkins,

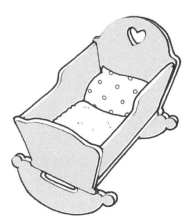

crazy games, even lawn furniture can make its way to the baby shower house.

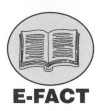

Virtual Shower Themes

Here are some virtual shower "seedlings" to get your party ideas flowing.

- ✓ **Grill Me Tender, Baby.** Fire up the grill, the best ribs are on the way! Mail order a load of barbequed ribs with all the fixin's, including sauce, corn bread, and coleslaw.
- ✓ **The Maine Event Lobster Bake.** Make Mom's mouth water when she opens the door to this portable lobster bake straight from the icy waters of the North Atlantic. She'll love the idea of wearing this bib, and so will her guests. Lobster bakes are available for two to twenty people, depending on your budget.
- ✓ **Let Them Eat Cake.** Or cookies. Or cheesecake. Send a phenomenal dessert. If you have a favorite bakery, ask them if they do mail order. If not, see what's recommended on the cooking shows or in a gourmand's magazine. See Appendix A for some sweet ideas.

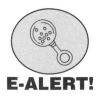

Gifts that Work with This Theme

If you are sending a gift to the home, size may not matter, but if the gift will arrive at a restaurant or other away-from-home location, you should consider the size of the mailing package as well as how the venue will store the gift until your shower date arrives. A canopy bassinette or baby carriage is sure to be appreciated, but its cumbersome arrival swathed in bubble-wrap and packing materials will make it difficult for a café to store and potentially impossible for the ride home.

✓ **Sterling silver.** Mail order from Tiffany's is more than a virtual gift, it's an actual keepsake. Consider a rattle, teething ring, handled cup, silver spoon, or even a silver toothbrush. And the boxes will fit in a purse.

✓ **Picture frames.** There will be plenty of pictures of the new baby, so there can't be too many frames. If you have old pictures of Mom or Dad you could also frame these and send them.

THEME IDEA 2	*The Desktop Shower: Coffee Break Contractions*

You can have a shower in fifteen minutes. That's what makes this idea perfect for the workplace, where fifteen minutes is about all the time you can spare. Commandeer a break room or meeting room to set up this speed shower, assign and delegate details and responsibilities, and send out an e-mail blast with date, place, and time.

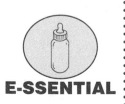

E-SSENTIAL

In larger offices, there is a continuous need to celebrate occasions—from birthdays to weddings to promotions to impending births. Sometimes it's hard to fit a workday into the mix! Get together with fellow workers and management to determine how these important, but often endless, celebrations will be handled. Some corporate cultures are tolerant of workplace parties, and others prefer that parties be held off-premise.

Invitation Ideas and Script

Send an e-mail or e-mail blast to those who will be invited to the fifteen-minute break. Here's a script:

Attention F.O.M. (Friend of Mother)!
As you can see, Haley is going to be a mom! We're going to celebrate at "Coffee-Break Contractions" on Tuesday, February 16th, at 10:15 A.M. in Room 216. Your department should bring a coffee cake for ten people, and we are chipping in $10 each for a baby stroller. Call or e-mail Beth with questions. See you Tuesday!

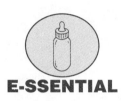

E-SSENTIAL

A workplace e-mail invitation might be the easiest way to get everyone on board for a shower, but check your office's policy regarding personal e-mails sent from work. It is also important to consider proper office etiquette—include the entire team and avoid the hurt feelings that come from being excluded, especially if the party will take place at work.

The Ultimate Coffee Break

Make the coffee break special by adding a touch of class to the regular brews and ordering in some fancy scones and biscotti to complete this morning break. If you can coordinate a coffee specialist or cart, this is the occasion for it; if not, bring in a custom-roasted blend from your local coffee company. For an afternoon breaktime shower, you could set up a "milk and cookies" bar. Give attendees a box of animal crackers with a tag that says "thank you" to take back to their desks.

Another option for the Ultimate Coffee Break is to rent a cappuccino cart. They can be rented by the hour and include a barista, coffee supplies, cleanup, and all drinks made-to-order during the hour. They can also provide breakfast pastries for an additional fee. Many companies that offer coffee carts also can make smoothies and other frozen concoctions, which are a great treat for the workplace in warm-weather months.

Setting It Up

When planning the coffee-break shower, the idea is to come in with display-ready items, rather than having to open bags and packages of supplies for complicated and time-consuming arrangements. Have an at-home run-through to avoid leaving behind a critical piece.

Organize what you need by category—table décor, food service, liquids, favors, and so on—and place in separate boxes or handled bags. Number the boxes (or bags) according to which should be used first. Table décor should be set up first, then food trays, beverage supplies, and, finally, gifts and favors. Enlist the help of coworkers to stage the party with speed and efficiency. Setup should take about fifteen minutes.

Many coffee-roasting companies have burlap bags that the raw beans come in that they sell or give away. These lend the right flavor to the table. Scrunch them up under trays or lay them over a tablecloth to add another layer. Coffee cans can be used to house a potted geranium or a bunch of colorful flowers (silk or fresh). If you are giving coffee-mug favors have them displayed as part of the décor—either in rows or on a mug tree.

Menu Ideas and Options

Here's one idea for an ultimate coffee-break menu:

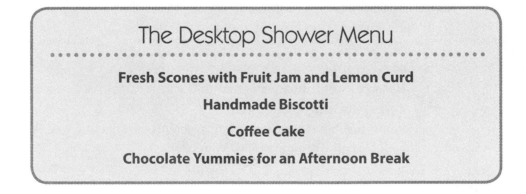

The Desktop Shower Menu

Fresh Scones with Fruit Jam and Lemon Curd

Handmade Biscotti

Coffee Cake

Chocolate Yummies for an Afternoon Break

Or you can tap your local coffee-roasting company for drink and food ideas or use the ideas listed here:

✓ **Breakfast fare.** Cream scones, handmade biscotti, and cinnamon coffee cake are easy to make and delicioso! (See Chapter 19 for these recipes.)

✓ **Syrups.** Torani syrups, a favorite beverage flavoring used at coffee houses, is available in most grocery stores. Choose three flavors from the most popular syrups, such as Amaretto, French Vanilla, Chocolate Milano, Almond Roca, Caramel, Hazelnut, and Irish Cream.

✓ **Toppers and touches.** Have a selection of toppers and touches including items like ground cinnamon, whole cloves, orange peel, cocoa powder, half-and-half, whipped cream, shaved chocolate, and nutmeg.

✓ **Novelty stirrers.** Dip plastic spoons in several coats of melted chocolate—dark, milk, and white. The chocolate melts in the coffee to create a delicious mocha confection. Substitute a peppermint stick submerged in milk chocolate to make the holiday season extra bright. Cinnamon sticks, sans chocolate, also make great stirrers and add a hint of European panache to the beverage.

Gifts that Work with This Theme

The workplace shower is the perfect place for a group gift. You can use the mom's gift registry as a guide for presents in your price range or purchase a gift certificate. Gift credit cards (Visa, Mastercard, and American Express are all available at the grocery store) are also options for giving a group gift that she can spend on the item she needs.

✓ **Jogging stroller.** For the athletic coworker mom.

✓ **Desk or "work" table.** Help mom create a "work" space for baby to play, draw, and create.

✓ **Photo printer.** These printers are exclusively for photos. They are small, relatively inexpensive, and portable.

Favors

Customized coffee mugs can be ordered in small batches or larger quantities if the workforce warrants it. Have some printed with a phrase or clip art or use the art work shown. Complete the favor with a themed message by attaching a shipping tag with a "Thanks a Latte" label. (See Appendix A.)

If the custom coffee mugs aren't your cup of tea, how about giving demitasse cups filled with chocolate-covered coffee beans? Tie the "Thanks a Latte" shipping tag to the top of the bean bag or on the handle of these tiny treats (see *www.everydayeventplanner.com*).

<table>
<tr><td>THEME IDEA 3</td><td>*The "Lap-Top" Shower Visit*</td></tr>
</table>

Mama is definitely getting a new "lap-top" accessory, the low-tech, high-maintenance kind that has a built-in no-sleep feature. If your favorite mom-to-be is now a mom-for-real, it's not too late to shower her with attention. Of course, this shower is more of a visit. The gift-giving advantage is that you know what gender the baby is and might have a good idea of what she needs, has, or still wants. The disadvantage is that her life, as well as her schedule, her sleep patterns, and her patience, have changed. A full-blown shower with all the trimmings may not be in the cards right now.

The "Lap-Top" Shower is the solution. It combines the speed of a pop-in visit with the gift-giving capacity of a shower, and it has the added benefit of Mommy getting to show off baby to boot.

Menu Ideas and Options

These recipes are easy to pack up and take out—to the exhausted new parents. Make a pan of one of the choices below and send with love and a loaf of French bread.

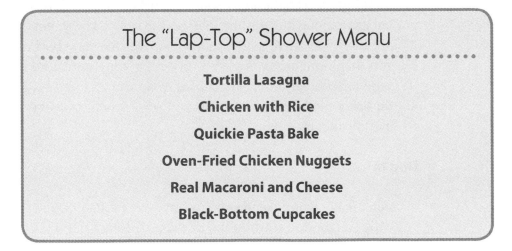

The "Lap-Top" Shower Menu

Tortilla Lasagna

Chicken with Rice

Quickie Pasta Bake

Oven-Fried Chicken Nuggets

Real Macaroni and Cheese

Black-Bottom Cupcakes

Setting It Up

The setup for this is simple: Call the new mom and find out when she has thirty minutes to see you. Emphasize flexibility and shortness of stay. In addition to any baby gift you plan to bring, consider a little something for the new parents to eat after you leave—dinner, a plate of cookies, or even a few comfort-food grocery items to save Mom a trip out.

Helping Hand Do's and Don'ts

New moms, especially brand-new mothers, don't always realize the daunting adjustments that are made during the first few weeks of parenthood. She will be forever grateful if you remember these simple rules:

Do's

✓ **Do ask.** Babies are so lovely to hold, but ask before you grab. Newborn moms may have a preferred way for you to pick up or handle their precious bundle. Be respectful of this new experience and be guided by her wishes.

✓ **Do help out.** Throw in a load of baby clothes, wash a sinkful of dishes, make up a batch of baby bottles, or offer to run an errand.

✓ **Do offer to watch baby.** Mom may not feel like going out, she may just want a hot shower or long nap. Give her an opportunity to get cleaned up and refreshed.

✓ **Do bring presents for older siblings.** This is not a strict requirement, but it is a thoughtful gesture that let's the sibling know that they have not been forgotten in the hullabaloo over the new baby. Crayons and a coloring book, a picture book, or some miniature cars can keep big brother or sister occupied while you visit.

✓ **Do bring food.** Dinner is great, and so is lunch, breakfast, or kid-friendly meals.

Don'ts

✓ **Don't make figure comments.** As any wise mother can tell you, the baby weight doesn't drop the day you deliver. It can be a stunning shock to many new moms that their prepregnancy clothes don't fit in the weeks after the birth.

✓ **Don't give unsolicited advice.** It may be tempting, and you may be right, but new moms want to learn on their own.

✓ **Don't eat the food.** If you have brought a meal, leave it for the new parents. There will be plenty of time down the road for dinner parties. Moms, dads, and babies need lots of extra rest and time to get to know each other.

✓ **Don't bring germs.** Even if it's just "allergies," keep sneezes, coughs, and runny noses away from baby. You will have a lifetime to visit. Make sure to wash your hands when you arrive at baby's house.

✓ **Don't overstay your welcome.** Moms and babies need rest. Unless you are babysitting, keep your visit short and sweet.

✓ **Don't bring other children.** Double-check with the new mom before you bring young children to visit baby for the first few times.

✓ **Don't bring a crowd.** Entertaining a crowd of adults can be overwhelming to a new mom who may be exhausted and whose house may not be as spiffed up and party ready as she would like it to be.

Gifts That Work with This Theme

In addition to the baby gifts that come with a first visit, there are a number of things that you can bring to help moms and dads make the transition to parenthood. During the first two weeks after baby is born, there are lots of hands ready to help. But as the next few weeks pass, the offers of help diminish and just about that time is when baby gets her second wind, so to speak. This is the time when a prepared meal that arrives on your doorstep along with an offer to watch the little napster while mom showers is a godsend.

Here are some practical ideas to take to the first visit:

✓ **Kid-friendly food basket.** If there are older siblings, their particular food likes may have been forgotten in the avalanche of meals that have arrived. Bring a box of kid-friendly foods like peanut butter, grape jelly, Ritz crackers, goldfish crackers, bread, bananas, juice boxes, pretzels, applesauce, mini-yogurts, frozen waffles, string cheese, cereal (Cheerios is always a safe bet), and milk.

✓ **Drugstore run.** Toilet paper, sanitizing soap, baby detergent, hand lotion, shampoo, infant Tylenol (check with mom first), and ChapStick.

✓ **Date night at-home basket.** For the many Saturday nights that will be spent at home, give mom and dad a six-month subscription to Netflicks or Blockbuster, bags of microwave popcorn, and a movie-trivia book.

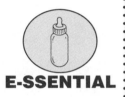

E-SSENTIAL

Polish the look of your gift basket by packing items in a useable container then enhancing with colored tissue paper, clear cellophane, and a big bow. Try using old-fashioned lunch boxes to deliver items in the kid-friendly food basket. Prop up contents with tissue, then envelop in cellophane so that the items can be seen. A Moses basket could be used to hold the treats for date night at home.

Celebrating a New Bundle of Joy

From the conception of a shower idea to the birth of the party, planning an event for a friend, neighbor, coworker, or family member is an undertaking that should be approached with a spirit of celebration. And anyone can deliver a great shower. You can set up a luncheon in your home or a scavenger hunt in your neighborhood. You can have an all-girl slumber party or an all-guy tailgating party, and both can be turned into baby showers. From an elegant red-carpet-style cocktail party to a Zen-inspired day of relaxation and henna tattoos to an extreme nursery makeover, the baby shower can be tailored to the interests, needs, and personal styles of Mom, Dad, and baby. If there's one thing that the ideas in this book demonstrate, it's that any party can be a baby shower. And any baby shower can be a bundle of fun.

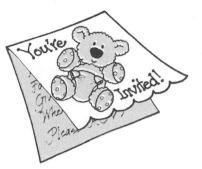

Chapter 19

Shower Recipes

FEEDING TIME IS just as critical at a shower as it is for the new baby. As shower traditions have changed, so too have shower menus. No longer the exclusive milieu for Jell-O molds and sugary cakes, the shower menu can be as varied as the guests and their tastes. Any food preference, recipe favorite, or tempting new trend can be the basis for a terrific shower menu. In this chapter, you will find some menus for three basic meals: the classic brunch, a ladies' lunch, and a couples' dinner, along with the recipes to make them. These menu plans can be used for any shower, regardless of theme.

Recipes and Ideas

So many recipes, so little time! Part of the fun of hosting is to spread your culinary wings and fly, but when the demands of real life—the juggling of kids, carpools, and work deadlines encroach—you can grab this section and head straight to the grocery store. The following recipes may inspire you to try something new, or allow you to substitute a family favorite for one of the dishes suggested. All the dishes have been prepared and served to real families who rated, reviewed, and applauded them. Be brave—have a trial run on your own family circle, then serve away.

The recipes that follow have been selected because they are: great tasting; easy to prepare; serve a crowd; can be prepared one to two days in advance (in most cases); can be adapted to suit your own taste and style; and can be adapted to different serving methods. All things necessary when throwing a shower!

Chapter 9: Celebrity-Style Baby Showers: Under Construction

Fourth of July–Ade (nonalcoholic)
Makes 20 Drinks

> 2 cups pomegranate juice
> 12 ounces pink-grapefruit juice
> 2 bottles of ginger ale

Mix all ingredients together and chill well.

Get Your Snack Mixer On
Serves 16

6 cups mixed cereal (such as unsweetened bran,
  oat, rice, and wheat cereal mix)
1 cup mini bow-knot pretzels
⅔ cup dry-roasted peanuts
⅛ cup (2 tablespoons) butter, melted
⅛ cup (2 tablespoons) olive, canola, or peanut oil
1 tablespoon Worcestershire sauce
¼ teaspoon garlic powder
Tabasco sauce or other liquid hot pepper sauce, to taste

1. Preheat oven to 300°F. In a large bowl, combine the cereal, pretzels, and peanuts. In another bowl, combine the butter, oil, Worcestershire, garlic powder,
   and Tabasco (if using).
2. Pour liquid ingredients over the cereal mixture and toss to coat evenly. Spread
   the mixture on a large baking sheet and bake for 30 to 40 minutes, stirring
   every 10 minutes, until crisp and dry.

Sirloin, Round, and Chuck Burger
Makes 8 Burgers

1 pound ground sirloin
1 pound ground chuck steak (not overly lean)
1 pound ground round
2 tablespoons of your favorite steak sauce or Worcestershire sauce
Salt and freshly ground black pepper to taste
8 slices tomato and/or sweet onion for garnish
Ketchup, mustard, and pickle relish to taste

1. Mix the three types of ground meat together, tossing lightly with steak sauce,
   salt, and pepper. Don't be heavy-handed here.
2. Preheat grill to medium-high.
3. Form burgers without too much patting and squeezing; this keeps them juicy.

4. Grill burgers over medium heat until they are nicely browned on the outside and pink on the inside, about 5 minutes per side. Timing depends on how thick the burgers are and how done you like them. Don't press the juice out with a spatula while cooking unless you like dry burgers.

5. Serve on hamburger buns, hard rolls, Portuguese rolls, or Tuscan bread with the toppings of your choice. Garnish with tomatoes and sweet onions.

Bright Chili Beans
Makes 2 Cups

½ cup vegetable oil
2 cloves garlic, peeled and minced
2 red onions, peeled and chopped
2 jalapeno peppers, cored and seeded
1 sweet red pepper, roasted, peeled, and chopped
1 (13-ounce) can red kidney beans or black beans
1 tablespoon Worcestershire sauce
1 teaspoon Tabasco sauce
1 tablespoon cocoa powder
6 ounces beer

1. Heat the oil in a large pot over medium-low heat. Add the garlic, onions, and peppers. Cook, stirring to soften the vegetables, 5 to 7 minutes.

2. Stir in the rest of the ingredients. Cover and cook for 4 to 5 hours. If it's too soupy, uncover and let the liquid cook out. Use as a topping for burgers.

German Potato Salad
Serves 8-12

3 pounds red bliss, fingerling, or creamery new potatoes
Cold water to cover with 2 tablespoons salt added
1½ cups red wine vinegar
1½ cups olive oil
2 red onions, peeled and sliced paper thin
2 teaspoons peppercorns, cracked
2 teaspoons caraway seeds, cracked
1 cup fresh parsley, rinsed and chopped

1. Scrub the potatoes but do not peel. Cut into bite-sized pieces. Put them in cold, salted water and bring to a boil. Boil potatoes for about 20 minutes, depending on size, until soft.
2. While the potatoes are cooking, mix the rest of the ingredients in a large serving bowl to make the dressing.
3. Drain the potatoes and mix them with the dressing. Serve hot, cold, or at room temperature.

Brownie Bar with Candy-Bar Toppings
Makes 16 squares

12 tablespoons unsalted butter, melted
1½ cups sugar
2 eggs
½ teaspoon vanilla extract
2 tablespoons water
¾ cup unsweetened cocoa powder
½ cup all-purpose flour
½ teaspoon salt
½ teaspoon baking powder
1 cup semisweet chocolate chips
1 large bag of mini candy bars or 6 to 8 regular-sized bars, chopped coarsely

1. Preheat oven to 350°F. Grease a 9" × 13" baking dish.
2. Mix together the butter and sugar in a mixing bowl.
3. Beat the eggs into the butter mixture, then stir in the vanilla and water.
4. In a separate bowl, combine the cocoa powder, flour, salt, and baking powder. Add this dry mixture to the wet mixture; stir to combine. Stir in the chocolate chips. Scrape the batter into the prepared baking dish, and smooth out the top of the batter.
5. Bake brownies for 30 minutes. Cool slightly in pan, top with chopped candy bars and cut into sixteen squares. Serve warm or at room temperature.

Chapter 9: Celebrity-Style Baby Showers: The Princess Wears Prada

These recipes were designed to be served in barwear—from appetizers in shot glasses to a main course in margarita glasses to dessert in demitasse cups. It's small bites but big flavor.

Rose Lemonade with Rose Petals
Serves 8

>   8 cups cold water
>   Juice of 4 large lemons
>   8 tablespoons sugar
>   2 teaspoons rose water

1. In a blender, blend all the ingredients until the sugar is dissolved.
2. Serve over crushed ice.

Minted Pea Soup
Makes 6 Cups, about 30 Shots

>   2 (10-ounce) packages frozen peas
>   2 cups water
>   2 14½-ounce cans chicken broth
>   Juice of 1 lemon
>   1 clove garlic, minced
>   1 small onion, chopped
>   Salt and pepper to taste
>   Small handful mint leaves, chopped
>   ¼ cup plain yogurt

1. Cook the peas in 2 cups of boiling water for just a few minutes. Drain, reserving water for use later in the recipe.
2. Puree the peas in a food processor. Mix 2 cups of the cooking water, broth, and lemon juice in a saucepan. Add the pureed peas and bring to a simmer. Add garlic, onion, salt, and pepper. Turn off heat. Add the mint to the soup. Serve with a dollop of yogurt.

Carrot and Parsnip with Ginger
Makes about 5 Cups, about 25 Shots

  3 cups shredded carrots
  3 cups shredded parsnips
  1" piece ginger root
  2 cups reduced-sodium, fat-free vegetable broth
  ¾ cup 2 percent milk
  1 teaspoon lemon juice
  Salt and white pepper

1. Shred the carrots, parsnips, and the peeled ginger root.
2. Using a soup pot, add the carrots, parsnips, ginger, and broth. Bring to a boil, reduce to a simmer, and cook for 25 minutes.
3. Remove from heat and allow to cool slightly. Using a blender or food processor, purée the soup. Add the milk and reheat almost to a boil. Add the lemon juice and salt and white pepper to taste.

Chilled Tomato Soup with Guacamole
Makes 6 Cups, about 30 Shots

1 leek	4 dried fennel sticks
1 stalk celery	1 tablespoon anise seeds
1 bulb fennel (small)	2 teaspoons fennel seeds
1 red bell pepper	1 teaspoon coriander seeds
½ Spanish onion	3 tablespoons olive oil
15 large beefsteak tomatoes	3 cups water
5 cloves garlic	White pepper to taste
1 sprig thyme	Tabasco sauce to taste
1 sprig rosemary	Celery salt (or onion salt)
3 sprigs parsley	4–6 tablespoons guacamole
2 sprigs basil	4–6 nasturtium flowers (optional)

1. Coarsely chop the leek (white part only). Coarsely chop the celery, fennel bulb, red bell pepper (discarding seeds and membranes), and the Spanish onion. Cut each of the tomatoes into eight pieces. Crush the garlic cloves gently.

2. Prepare two bouquet garnis: In the first bag, combine the thyme, rosemary, parsley, basil, and fennel sticks. In the second bag, combine the anise, fennel, and coriander seeds.
3. In a soup pot, heat the olive oil. Add the leek, celery, fennel bulb, red bell pepper, onion, and garlic. Cover, turn the heat very low, and allow to soften for 10 minutes.
4. Add the two bouquet garnis, the tomato pieces, and the water. Bring to a boil, reduce to a simmer, and cook for 15 minutes.
5. Remove from heat and allow to cool slightly. Discard the bouquet garnis. Using a blender or food processor, puree the mixture. Season with salt, white pepper, Tabasco sauce, and celery salt to taste. Refrigerate to chill thoroughly.
6. Ladle the soup into individual serving bowls. Garnish each with 1 tablespoon of guacamole and a nasturtium flower.

Garden-Pea Couscous Salad with Roasted Chicken Breast
Serves 8

2 pounds roasted boneless, skinless chicken breast, diced
1½ cups couscous
1½ cups chicken broth
1 tablespoon olive oil
2 cups frozen peas
2 large bunches of fresh mint, finely chopped
Juice of 4 lemons
2 tablespoons of lemon zest
Salt and pepper to taste

1. In a large saucepan, bring chicken broth and olive oil to a boil. When liquid is at a rolling boil, remove from heat.
2. Immediately add couscous, cover, and leave standing for 5 minutes.
3. Place peas in a strainer and run under warm water to thaw. Drain and set aside.
4. When couscous has cooled slightly, mix in peas, lemon juice, salt, and pepper.
5. Once couscous mixture has cooled to room temperature, mix in chopped mint, lemon zest, and diced chicken. Serve at room temperature in margarita glasses and garnish with a lemon wheel.

Parmesan Crisps
Makes 40 Crisps

1 loaf French bread baguette (about 12")
1 cup butter
1 cup grated Parmesan cheese

1. Preheat oven to 400°F.
2. Slice the baguette into ¼" slices, discarding the heels. In a small flat-bottomed baking dish, melt the butter. In a similar bowl, place the grated cheese. Quickly dip each side of the bread slices in butter (do not soak!), then in the cheese. Place in a jellyroll pan (do not substitute a cookie sheet because some butter may drain off in cooking).
3. Bake 5 minutes, then turn slices over. Bake an additional 4 minutes or until browned.

Coffee-Almond Float in Espresso Cups
Makes 16

4 teaspoons brown sugar
4 cups brewed cold coffee
4–6 teaspoons of orgeat (almond syrup)
Ice cubes
8 cups 1 percent milk
6 cups coffee or chocolate low-fat frozen yogurt

In a demitasse glass cup, dissolve the sugar in the coffee. Add the syrup, stirring to mix well. Add the ice and milk and stir well. Top with the frozen yogurt.

Chocolate Shortbread
Serves 12

1 cup butter
1 cup confectioners' sugar
2 cups all-purpose flour
Pinch of salt
1 tablespoon vanilla extract
3 ounces bittersweet chocolate, melted
3 tablespoons white or turbinado sugar

1. With a hand-held mixer, cream together butter and confectioners' sugar until light and fluffy.
2. Whisk together salt and flour, stirring to break up any lumps in the mixture. Slowly stir flour into the butter and sugar. Stir in vanilla and melted chocolate and mix until blended.
3. Roll mixture into a ball, wrap in plastic wrap, and refrigerate for 1 hour.
4. Spread mixture onto waxed paper and cut into 2 dozen large cookies, using a heart or circle-shaped cookie cutter. Sprinkle each cookie with sugar and place on a greased cookie sheet. Bake at 300°F for 15–20 minutes.

Chapter 9: Celebrity-Style Baby Showers: Roll Out the Red Carpet

Eggplant Caviar
Makes 2 Cups

1 cup finely chopped onion
1 cup finely chopped bell pepper
2 tablespoons olive oil
1 large eggplant, cooked and innards scooped out and mashed
1 tomato, finely chopped
Salt and pepper to taste

1. In a large skillet, brown the onion and green pepper in the olive oil. Add eggplant and tomato and stir often. Cook until the mixture is well done. Add more oil if it begins to stick. Add salt and pepper to taste. Transfer the mixture to a serving dish and chill.
2. Serve as a spread for crackers or as a vegetable dip.

Herb-Crusted Salmon
Serves 8

8 6-ounce salmon steaks
Salt and freshly ground black pepper to taste
2 egg whites, well beaten
Juice of 1 lemon
Zest of 1 lemon
4 tablespoons fresh parsley, chopped
2 tablespoons fresh dill, chopped
2 teaspoons dried oregano

1. Rinse the salmon in cold water and pat dry on paper towels. Sprinkle the salmon with salt and pepper. Paint the salmon on both sides with the egg white.
2. Mix the rest of the ingredients together and press them into the fish. Let stand for a few minutes.
3. Heat the grill to medium-low.
4. Grill the salmon slowly for about 4–5 minutes per side, depending on the thickness.

Stuffed Filet Mignon
Serves 8

4 garlic cloves, minced
4 shallots, minced
1½ cups chopped mushrooms
¾ cup melted butter or olive oil
1 cup soft breadcrumbs
Salt and pepper to taste
4 tablespoons parsley, finely chopped
1 teaspoon red pepper flakes (optional)
8 very thick filet mignons
8 wooden toothpicks, soaked for 1 hour in water

1. Sauté the garlic, shallots, and mushrooms in the butter or oil over low heat for 10 minutes.
2. Add the breadcrumbs, salt, pepper, parsley, and red pepper flakes.

3. Cut slits in the side of each filet. Divide the stuffing among the filets and press into the "pockets." (At this point, you can refrigerate for up to 8 hours.)
4. Prepare the grill to medium-high.
5. Grill the filets for 5 minutes per side, then let them rest. Sauce and serve.

Classic Asparagus with Lemon and Olive Oil
Serves 8

> 2 pounds asparagus
> 1 cup olive oil
> Juice of 1 lemon

1. Rinse the asparagus and pat dry on paper towels. Remove the tough, woody bottoms. Using a vegetable peeler, remove tough outer skin, starting halfway down the spears.
2. Set grill for medium-low and make room for indirect heat.
3. Using thin metal skewers of about 12 inches in length, skewer the asparagus across the bottom and again, halfway up. Sprinkle with oil and lemon juice.
4. Grill for about 8–10 minutes per side, depending on the heat of the grill and the thickness of the spears. Serve with lemon butter.

Yukon Gold Potatoes with Oregano
Serves 8

> 8 Yukon Gold potatoes, scrubbed
> 8 tablespoons olive oil
> 8 teaspoons dried oregano
> Salt and pepper to taste

1. Set the grill to medium.
2. Cut the potatoes in quarters, lengthwise, and place on a piece of heavy-duty aluminum foil.
3. Drizzle with olive oil and sprinkle with oregano, salt, and pepper.
4. Place on grill, lid closed, and let bake for 20 minutes; check often. They're done when the outside is brown and crunchy and the inside is soft.

Grilled Pears with Claret Sauce
Serves 8

2 cups claret
4 whole cloves, bruised
½ cup sugar (optional)
½ cup heavy cream
8 unpeeled pears, halved and cored

1. Bring the claret, cloves, and sugar to a boil and reduce to half. Add the cream and keep warm.
2. Set grill to high heat.
3. Grill the pears over a hot fire for 1 minute, cut-side down. Turn and grill for 30 seconds. Remove pears to serving plates, spoon sauce over all, and serve immediately.

Chocolate Butter-Rum Truffles
Makes 5 Dozen

1 cup heavy cream
⅓ cup sugar
Pinch of salt
1 teaspoon vanilla
½ pound high-quality dark chocolate
½ pound high-quality milk chocolate
1¼ cups unsalted butter
3 tablespoons dark rum or 1 teaspoon rum extract
Choice of chocolate fondue for dipping
Confectioners' sugar for coating

1. Combine cream, sugar, salt, and vanilla in a medium saucepan. Bring mixture to a boil, stirring often. Finely chop dark and milk chocolate. Remove cream mixture from heat and stir in chopped chocolate. Stir resulting ganache until melted and smooth.
2. Pour chocolate ganache into a glass mixing bowl and allow to cool. Cream butter with dark rum or rum extract. Whisk into chocolate ganache a spoonful at a time until mixture is creamy and well blended.

3. Spoon small dollops of mixture onto a baking sheet lined with waxed paper. Or, place mixture in a pastry bag and pipe balls of ganache onto the sheet. Refrigerate for at least 2 hours or until centers have hardened.

4. Using a wooden skewer or fondue forks, dip the centers into chocolate fondue to coat. Allow excess chocolate to drip off, then roll truffle in the confectioners' sugar and set on wax-paper–lined baking sheet to set. Keep truffles cool until ready to package or serve.

Espresso Truffles
Makes 5 Dozen

⅔ cup cream
⅔ cup sugar
2 tablespoons espresso powder or instant coffee
3 tablespoons corn syrup
1 pound good-quality dark chocolate
1 teaspoon vanilla
1¼ cups unsalted butter
Choice of chocolate fondue for dipping
Mixture of cocoa powder and espresso powder (2 to 1) for coating

1. In a medium saucepan, bring cream and sugar to a boil, stirring constantly. Whisk in espresso or coffee powder, and stir until dissolved. Whisk in corn syrup. Remove cream from heat. Finely chop chocolate and add to hot cream a small amount at a time, stirring until completely melted.

2. Cool chocolate-coffee mixture completely. In a large bowl, cream softened butter with vanilla. Slowly whisk cooled chocolate-coffee into butter mixture until smooth and creamy.

3. Using a spoon or a pastry bag, place dollops of chocolate-coffee mixture onto a parchment- or waxed-paper–lined baking sheet. Refrigerate until hardened, at least ¼ hour.

4. Using fondue or wooden skewers, dip truffle centers into dark or light chocolate fondue. Combine cocoa and espresso. Roll dipped truffles into powder mixture and place on a baking sheet. Keep cool until ready to package or serve.

Chapter 10: Girlfriends Go Wild Shower: Playing Footsie, Tootsie!

Strawberry Lemonade
Makes 5 Cups

¾ cup fresh-squeezed lemon juice
½ cup sugar
4 cups water
½ cup fresh strawberries, hulled and sliced
Ice cubes

1. Purée strawberries in the blender or food processor.
2. Combine lemon juice, sugar, and water, then stir in strawberry puree. Serve over ice.

Salad Bar

Simply pick a few favorites from the list of suggested ingredients and serve. Select two lettuces and one or two ingredients from each category to offer guests an enticing array for their plate.

✓ **Lettuces:** romaine, butter lettuce, iceberg, field greens, lamb's lettuce, spinach, micro-greens
✓ **Dried fruit:** cranberries, cherries, apricots, and papaya
✓ **Fresh fruits:** grapes, apples, pears, avocado, sun-dried tomatoes, cherry tomatoes, oranges, and pomegranate seeds
✓ **Nuts and seeds:** Glazed walnuts or pecans, slivered almonds, toasted pine nuts, sunflower seeds, or sesame seeds
✓ **Vegetables:** shredded carrots, jicama, cucumber, peas, radishes, scallions, red onions, corn, beets, peppers (red, yellow, and green), olives, green beans, capers, pickles
✓ **Beans and grains:** Taboule, garbanzo beans, kidney beans, cannellini (white beans), black beans, barley, quinoa, alfalfa sprouts, bamboo shoots

- ✓ **Meats and fish:** smoked turkey, ham, bacon, shredded chicken, grilled chicken breast, steak, shrimp, tuna, salmon
- ✓ **Cheeses:** shredded or shaved Parmesan, feta cheese, goat cheese, fresh mozzarella, Cheddar (cubed or grated), blue cheese, Gorgonzola
- ✓ **Crunchies:** French-bread croutons, rice noodles, tortilla strips, Parmesan crisps
- ✓ **Dressings:** Ranch, balsamic vinaigrette, Caesar, honey mustard, champagne vinaigrette

Texas Sheet Cake
Serves 12

2 cups all-purpose flour
2 cups sugar
½ teaspoon salt
1 stick butter
½ cup vegetable shortening
1 cup water
6 tablespoons cocoa powder
½ cup sour cream
2 eggs
1 teaspoon vanilla extract
Dash of cinnamon
1 teaspoon baking soda

1. Combine flour, sugar, and salt in a bowl. Stir with a whisk to blend and break up any lumps.
2. In a large saucepan, combine butter, shortening, water, and cocoa powder. Cook, stirring, over medium-high heat until mixture comes to a boil. Remove from heat and let cool until just warm.
3. Pour cocoa mixture over flour and sugar. Beat with a mixer until smooth. Add sour cream, eggs, vanilla, cinnamon, and baking soda. Mix well. Pour into a buttered 11" × 16" sheet pan and bake at 350°F for 20 minutes.
4. When cake is halfway done, make frosting. Melt butter, cocoa, and milk in a saucepan over medium heat. Bring to a boil and remove from heat. Add confectioners' sugar, vanilla, and pecans. Mix until blended.
5. Pour frosting over hot cake and carefully smooth over the top. Cool and serve.

Chapter 10: Girlfriends Go Wild Shower: Cute as a Button

Pink Ladies'-Ade
Serves 8

1 box frozen raspberries, defrosted

1 small can frozen lemonade, mixed with 2 cans water

1 bottle pink champagne

1 bottle regular brut champagne (or club soda)

1 pint fresh strawberries, washed, hulled, and halved

20 fresh mint leaves

Whirl the raspberries and lemonade in your blender until pureed. Place in a punch bowl. Add the rest of the ingredients and mix gently.

Smoked Turkey Salad
Serves 8

2 pounds of smoked turkey; have the deli cut it in ½" slices, then cube it at home

2 large heads of butter lettuce, washed and drained

¾ cup of glazed pecans or walnuts

½ cup of dried apricots, chopped

½ cup dried cranberries

½ cup blue or Gorgonzola cheese, crumbled

1 bottle of Champagne salad dressing or other light-flavored vinaigrette

1. Tear lettuce into pieces and place in salad bowl.
2. Add remaining ingredients and toss together.
3. Just before serving, dress salad with vinaigrette.

Chapter 10: Girlfriends Go Wild Shower: Everything Night-Night

- -

Mexican Hot Chocolate
Serves 6–8

3 ounces unsweetened chocolate
½ cup white granulated sugar
2 tablespoons instant coffee
2 teaspoons ground cinnamon
1 teaspoon ground nutmeg
¼ teaspoon salt
2 cups water
4 cups whole milk
Whipped Cream

1. Place the chocolate, sugar, coffee, cinnamon, nutmeg, salt, and water in a large saucepan and heat over low heat until the chocolate melts and the mixture is smooth.
2. Bring to a boil. Turn heat to low and simmer for 5 minutes, stirring constantly. Stir in the milk. Beat with a hand beater until foamy.
3. Top with a dollop of whipped cream.

- -

Cookie-Cutter French Toast
Serves 8

12 eggs
3 cups milk
2 teaspoons vanilla extract
1 teaspoon cinnamon
16 tablespoons butter
16 slices day-old bread
½ cup powdered sugar

1. Combine eggs, milk, vanilla, and cinnamon in a shallow, flat bowl (like a soup or pasta bowl), using a whisk. Melt butter in a frying pan over medium heat, being careful not to let it burn.
2. Dip both sides of each slice of bread in the custard mixture and immediately pan-fry in melted butter on both sides.
3. Cut French toast with large cookie cutter (heart, baby carriage, etc.) and sprinkle with powdered sugar.
4. Serve with butter and warm maple syrup.

Crustless Quiche Lorraine
Serves 6–8

12 slices bacon
2 medium onions
3 tablespoons cooking oil
12 eggs
3 cups shredded Swiss cheese or a mixture of Swiss and Gruyere cheese
Dash nutmeg
Salt and pepper to taste

1. Preheat the broiler. Cook the bacon in a skillet until hard. Drain well, crumble, and reserve. Slice the onion very thinly. In a 10" ovenproof skillet, heat the oil and sauté the onion for about 2 minutes.
2. Beat the eggs well. Stir in the cheese, nutmeg, salt and pepper, and bacon. When the onions have finished cooking, stir to distribute evenly (do not drain), and pour the egg mixture over them. Reduce the heat to medium-low and cook until set but still moist on top, about 8 minutes. Immediately put the skillet in the broiler, about 5" from the flame or element, and cook until the top is done but not browned.

Chapter 11: Zen Tea Shower: Tranquili-Tea

Miso-Soup Shots
Makes 4 Cups

6 tablespoons miso paste (any kind)
4 cups water or dashi
½ cup (4 ounces) tofu, cut into ¼" cubes
1 scallion, sliced diagonally into ½" pieces

Bring the water (or dashi) almost to a boil in a saucepan; do not let it boil. Add the miso paste and the tofu pieces. Garnish with slices of scallion.

Cilantro Chicken Dumplings
Serves 8

16 wonton wrappers
1 cup chicken, finely minced or ground
⅓ cup cilantro, minced
1 green onion, minced
1 tablespoon soy sauce
1 tablespoon ginger, grated
2 tablespoons sesame oil
2 tablespoons white wine or broth
Salt and pepper to taste

1. Lay out half of the wonton wrappers on a cookie sheet and cover with waxed paper.
2. Combine chicken and remaining ingredients in a bowl. Mix lightly with fingers until blended. Place a generous tablespoon of chicken mixture into the center of each wonton wrapper. Wet edges together to seal. Trim edges to achieve half-moon shape. Repeat with remaining wonton wrappers.
3. Bring a pot of water to a boil. Add a few dumplings at a time to the pot, then reduce heat to simmering. Cook for 5–7 minutes or until dumplings turn translucent. With a slotted spoon, remove to a bowl and set aside. Dumplings will be warmed in fondue bowls.

Shrimp and Green-Onion Dumplings
Serves 8

1 cup shrimp, finely chopped
½ cup Chinese cabbage, minced
2 green onions, minced
2 tablespoons soy sauce
1 teaspoon sesame oil
2 cloves garlic, minced
2 tablespoons wine or broth
Salt and pepper to taste

1. Combine all ingredients in a bowl. Mix lightly with fingers until thoroughly combined.
2. Place a generous tablespoon of shrimp mixture into the center of each wonton wrapper. Wet edges of wrappers. Fold wrappers over filling diagonally and press edges together to seal. Trim edges to achieve half-moon shape. Repeat with remaining wonton wrappers.
3. Bring a pot of water to a boil. Add a few dumplings at a time to the pot, then reduce heat to simmering. Cook for 5–7 minutes or until dumplings turn translucent. With a slotted spoon, remove to a bowl and set aside. Dumplings will be warmed in fondue bowls.

Spring Rolls
Yields 12 Rolls

½ pound pork tenderloin, shredded
2 tablespoons oyster sauce, divided
6 dried mushrooms
1 carrot
1 tablespoon chicken broth or stock
½ teaspoon sugar
1 cup mung bean sprouts, rinsed and drained
2 green onions, thinly sliced on the diagonal
¼ teaspoon sesame oil
12 spring-roll wrappers
2 tablespoons plus ½ teaspoon cornstarch, divided
4–6 cups oil, for frying

1. Marinate the pork in 1 tablespoon oyster sauce and ½ teaspoon cornstarch for 30 minutes.
2. Soak the dried mushrooms in hot water to soften; drain and thinly slice. Wash and grate the carrot until you have ¼ cup.
3. Combine the remaining 1 tablespoon oyster sauce, chicken broth, and sugar. Set aside.
4. Add 2 tablespoons oil to a preheated wok or skillet. When oil is hot, add the pork. Stir-fry briefly until it changes color and is nearly cooked through. Remove from the wok.
5. Add 1½ tablespoons oil. When oil is hot, add the dried mushrooms. Stir-fry for 1 minute, then add the bean sprouts, grated carrot, and the green onion. Add the sauce in the middle of the wok and bring to a boil. Add the pork and mix through. Drizzle with the sesame oil. Cool.
6. Heat 4–6 cups oil to 375°F. While oil is heating, prepare the spring rolls. To wrap, lay the wrapper in a diamond shape. Place a tablespoon of filling in the middle. Coat all the edges with the cornstarch-and-water mixture. Roll up the wrapper and tuck in the edges. Seal the tucked-in edges with cornstarch and water. Continue with the remainder of the Spring Rolls. (Prepare more cornstarch and water as necessary.)
7. Deep-fry the spring rolls, 2 at a time, until they turn golden. Drain on paper towels.

Fried Bowties
Yields 2 Bowties for Every Wrapper

1 package egg-roll wrappers
¼ cup powdered sugar
Oil for deep-frying

1. Cut each wrapper vertically into 4 equal pieces. Cut a ¾" slit in the middle.
2. Take 2 long pieces and lay one piece on top of the other, then carefully tie a knot in the middle using both pieces. Your slits should end up in the knot. Starting with one side, tuck the two ends into the slit, then turn over and repeat with the other side. You should now have something that looks like a bow tie.
3. Heat 1½" of oil in a heavy skillet. Deep-fry a few of the bowties at a time until they are golden brown, turning over once. Remove from the pan with a slotted spoon and drain on paper towels.
4. Cool the bow ties and dust lightly with powdered sugar. Store in an airtight container. Serve cold.

Chapter 11: Zen Tea Shower: Belly Bump

Chai Tea Mix
Makes 4 Cups

  2 cups dry milk powder
  1 cup powdered nondairy creamer
  2 tablespoons vanilla powder
  2½ cups white sugar
  1½ cups unsweetened instant tea
  2 teaspoons ground ginger
  2 teaspoons ground cinnamon
  1 teaspoon ground cloves
  1 teaspoon ground nutmeg
  1 teaspoon ground cardamom

1. Combine milk powder, nondairy creamer, vanilla powder, sugar, and instant tea with ginger, cinnamon, cloves, nutmeg, and cardamom.
2. Stir 2 heaping tablespoons each of the tea mixture into mugs of hot water.

Saffron Lemonade
Serves 8

  8 cups cold water
  Juice of 8 large lemons
  12 tablespoons sugar or to taste
  1 teaspoon crushed saffron threads
  Fresh mint and lemon slices, for garnish

1. In a blender, blend together all the ingredients except the garnishes until the sugar is dissolved. Serve garnished with mint leaves and lemon slices.

Chicken Curry
Serves 8–10

6 tablespoons vegetable oil
2 black cardamom pods
4 green cardamom pods, bruised
4 cloves
2 (1") cinnamon sticks
2 bay leaves
2 large red onions, finely chopped
2 tablespoons Ginger-Garlic Paste
     (page 245)
4 medium tomatoes, finely chopped
1 teaspoon red chili powder

2 teaspoons Warm Spice Mix
     (page 245) plus extra for garnish
½ teaspoon turmeric powder
4 teaspoons coriander powder
Table salt, to taste
1 cup plain yogurt, whipped
5 pounds skinless chicken pieces,
     cuts of your choice
Water, as needed
4 tablespoons minced cilantro

1. In a large skillet, heat the oil on medium. Add the cardamom, cloves, cinnamon sticks, and bay leaves. When the spices begin to sizzle, add the onion and the Ginger-Garlic Paste. Sauté for about 5–7 minutes or until the onion is well browned.
2. Add the tomatoes to cook for about 8 minutes or until the tomatoes are soft and the oil begins to separate from the sides of the mixture.
3. Add the red chili powder, the spice mix, turmeric powder, coriander powder, and salt; cook for 1 minute. Add the yogurt and mix well. Cook, stirring constantly for 1 more minute.
4. Add the chicken and cook, stirring constantly for 5–7 minutes or until brown on all sides. Add 1 cup of water, cover, and simmer for 20 minutes or until the chicken is cooked through. Stir occasionally, and add more water if the sauce dries up or if you want a thinner gravy. Add the minced cilantro and cook for 1 minute. Serve hot, sprinkled with Warm Spice Mix.

Warm Spice Mix
Makes 2 Tablespoons

8 cloves
4 teaspoons cumin seeds
3 green cardamom pods (whole)
2 black cardamom pods (whole)
1 (2") cinnamon stick
2 teaspoons coriander seeds
1 teaspoon black peppercorns
1 bay leaf
Pinch of grated nutmeg (optional)

1. Heat a small skillet on medium. Add all the spices except the nutmeg and dry roast the spices, stirring constantly. After about 5 minutes, the spices will darken and begin to release a unique aroma.
2. Remove the skillet from the heat, then add the nutmeg. Transfer the spice mix to a bowl and allow to cool for about 5 minutes.
3. Using a spice grinder, grind the spices to a fine powder. Store in an airtight jar. The spice mixture will keep for up to three months.

Ginger-Garlic Paste
Makes 1 Cup

2 serrano green chilies (optional)
½ cup fresh gingerroot, peeled
½ cup garlic cloves, peeled
1 tablespoon cold water

1. Remove the stems from the green chilies.
2. Place all the ingredients in a food processor and purée for a smooth paste. Add no more than 1 tablespoon of water to help form a smooth consistency.
3. Store the paste in an airtight jar in the refrigerator. The paste will keep for up to two weeks in the refrigerator.

Malabari Coconut Rice
Serves 8–10

3 cups basmati rice
9 tablespoons vegetable oil
3 teaspoons black mustard seeds
6 dried red chilies, broken
6" piece fresh gingerroot, julienned
12 garlic cloves, minced

1½ teaspoons turmeric powder
Table salt, to taste
1½ cups unsweetened desiccated coconut
1½ cups light coconut milk
4½ cups water

1. Rinse the rice at least 3–4 times in water. Drain and set aside.
2. In a deep pan, heat the vegetable oil. Add the mustard seeds. When they begin to sputter, add the red chilies, ginger, and garlic; sauté for about 30 seconds.
3. Add the turmeric, salt, and coconut. Mix well and sauté for 1 minute. Add the rice and mix well; sauté for 1 minute.
4. Add the coconut milk and the water; stir for 1 minute. Bring to a boil.
5. Reduce the heat. Loosely cover the rice with a lid and cook for about 12–15 minutes or until most of the water has evaporated. You will see small craters forming on top of the rice.
6. Cover tightly and reduce the heat to the lowest setting; simmer for another 5–6 minutes.
7. Remove from heat and let stand, covered, for about 5 minutes. Fluff with a fork before serving.

Dry-Spiced Carrots and Peas
Serves 8–10

4 tablespoons vegetable oil
2 teaspoons cumin seeds
4 medium carrots (fresh or frozen), peeled and diced
4 cups peas (fresh or frozen)
1 teaspoon red chili powder
½ teaspoon turmeric powder
2 teaspoons coriander powder
Table salt, to taste
Water, as needed

1. In a medium-sized skillet, heat the vegetable oil over high heat. Add the cumin seeds. When the seeds begin to sizzle, add the carrots and peas; sauté for about 2 minutes.
2. Add the dry spices and salt, and mix well; sauté for about 2 minutes (if the dry spices begin to stick, add a few tablespoons of water).
3. Reduce the heat and add 2–3 tablespoons of water to the skillet. Cover and cook for about 15 minutes or until the carrots and peas are cooked. Serve hot.

Pomegranate Chaat
Serves 8-10

½ cup fresh raspberries	2 tablespoons fresh lemon juice
½ cup seedless grapes	2 tablespoons chopped cilantro
2 cups fresh pomegranate seeds	1 teaspoon cumin
½ cup fresh blueberries	2 teaspoons dried mint
½ cup canned mandarin oranges, drained	1 teaspoon ginger powder

Rinse the fresh berries in cool water and drain. Mix together all the ingredients in a bowl. Toss to evenly coat the fruits with the spices. Chill for about 20 minutes.

Chapter 12: A Grandparents' Shower

Stonepine Iced Tea
Makes 8 Cups

8 cups boiling water	1 cup honey
6 Orange Pekoe tea bags	4 oranges, thinly sliced
6 English Breakfast tea bags	20 fresh mint leaves, crushed

1. Pour boiling water over tea bags in a large bowl or heat-resistant pitcher. Allow to brew for 5–8 minutes, remove tea bags.
2. Stir in honey until dissolved, then let cool to room temperature.
3. Add sliced oranges and crushed mint. Serve over ice.

Grandma's Beef Stew
Serves 8

⅓ cup flour
1 teaspoon salt
¼ teaspoon freshly ground
    black pepper
2 pounds stewing beef, cut into cubes
¼ cup shortening
4 cups water
1 tablespoon lemon juice

1 tablespoon Worcestershire sauce
1 teaspoon sugar
1 large onion, sliced
2 bay leaves
¼ teaspoon allspice
12 small carrots, trimmed and scraped
12 small white onions, trimmed
8 small new potatoes, peeled

1. Mix together the flour, salt, and pepper. Toss the beef cubes in the mixture.
2. In a soup pot, melt the shortening on high heat. When the fat is very hot, add as many of the beef cubes to the pan as you can without crowding them, and brown on all sides; remove with a slotted spoon and set aside; repeat this process until all the beef is browned.
3. In a saucepan, bring the water to a boil. Return all the meat to the pot and add the boiling water. Stir in the lemon juice, Worcestershire sauce, sugar, onion, bay leaves, and allspice. Reduce the heat, cover, and simmer 1½–2 hours, until the meat is tender.
4. Add the carrots, onions, and potatoes; cover and cook 20–25 minutes, until the vegetables can be pierced easily with a fork. Discard the bay leaves.

Caesar Salad
Serves 8

3 tablespoons extra-virgin olive oil
2 tablespoons mayonnaise
Juice of ½ lemon
1 teaspoon anchovy paste
1 teaspoon Worcestershire sauce
1 teaspoon Dijon Mustard

¼ teaspoon coarsely ground
    black pepper
2 heads romaine lettuce, washed,
    dried, and torn into bite-size pieces
½ cup grated Parmesan cheese
1 10-ounce package thick croutons

Pour olive oil into a large wooden salad bowl. Add mayonnaise, lemon juice, anchovy paste, Worcestershire sauce, mustard, and pepper. Stir with a fork until will blended. Add lettuce and toss well to coat evenly with dressing. Add cheese and croutons and toss again.

Garlic Bread
Serves 8

2 loaves French bread
½ cup virgin olive oil
8 cloves garlic, minced
Freshly ground pepper to taste
½ teaspoon onion salt
3 tablespoons butter, melted
2 teaspoons chopped fresh or dried parsley

1. Preheat the grill. Slice the bread into 1" slices without cutting all the way to the bottom of each slice.
2. Combine the remaining ingredients in a mixing bowl and stir well. Using a basting brush, apply to both sides of the bread slices without separating the slices too far. Wrap the entire loaf in aluminum foil and set on the grill. Flip over after 4–6 minutes and heat for another 4–6 minutes.

Estelle's Cream-Cheese Pound Cake
Serves 8–12

1½ cups butter
3 cups sugar
1 8-ounce package cream cheese
6 eggs
1 teaspoon vanilla
3 cups cake flour
Powdered sugar

1. Preheat oven to 300°F. Grease a Bundt pan well.
2. Cream together the butter, sugar, and cream cheese until light and fluffy. Add the eggs one at a time, beating well after each, then add the vanilla. Add the flour slowly. Bake in the Bundt pan for 1½ hours.
3. Dust with sifted powdered sugar before serving. Cake may be served when cooked, but is even better the second day.

Raspberry Coulis
Serves 8–12

1 cup sugar
½ cup water
4 cups fresh or frozen raspberries

1. Dissolve sugar in water over low heat in a saucepan. Cool completely.
2. Purée raspberries in a blender, then strain into a bowl.
3. Combine raspberry puree with chilled sugar syrup.

Chapter 13: Broadway Baby Shower

Classic Swiss Cheese Fondue
Serves 12

3 pounds Gruyère cheese
2 loaves French bread
2 garlic cloves
3 cups dry white wine
2 tablespoons lemon juice

4 tablespoons cornstarch
6 tablespoons kirsch
¼ teaspoon cayenne pepper
2 tablespoons caraway seeds

1. Finely dice the Gruyère cheese and set aside. Cut the French bread into cubes and set aside.
2. Smash the garlic, peel, and cut in half. Rub the garlic around the inside of a medium saucepan. Discard. Add the wine to the saucepan and warm on medium-low heat. Don't allow the wine to boil.
3. When the wine is warm, stir in the lemon juice. Add the cheese, a handful at a time. Stir the cheese continually in a sideways figure-eight pattern. Wait until the cheese is completely melted before adding more. Don't allow the fondue mixture to boil.
4. When the cheese is melted, dissolve the cornstarch in the kirsch and add to the cheese, stirring. Turn up the heat until it is just bubbling and starting to thicken. Stir in the cayenne pepper and caraway seeds. Transfer to a fondue pot and set on the burner. Serve with the French bread for dipping or add dippers like vegetables, fresh fruits, or meats such as cooked sausages for a more interesting and substantial offering.

Chocolate Fondue
Serves 8

12-ounce bag semisweet chocolate chips
1 pint heavy cream

Assortment of dippers such as:
Fresh fruits, such as strawberries, pineapple, pears, bing cherries, and bananas
Dried fruits, such as apricots, mango, and papaya
Cakes, such as pound cake, angel cake, lady fingers, and brownies
Candy and Cookies, such as Snickers, gummy bears, Lorna Doones, marsh-
    mallows, Rice Krispie Treats, pretzels, and graham crackers

1. Melt cream and chocolate chips together in electric fondue pot, stirring constantly until blended. If using a flame-top fondue pot, melt cream and chocolate in a double–boiler, then transfer to pot.
2. Cut dippers into 1" cubes and arrange on trays and bowls. Use long skewers or fondue forks to dip.

Helen's Dulce de Leche Fondue
Serves 8

3 (14-ounce) cans sweetened condensed milk
Water for cooking

1. The Dulce de Leche is cooked in the unopened, unpunctured cans of sweetened, condensed milk. Be sure to remove the label from the cans.
2. Then stand cans in a saucepan and cover them with water. Bring the water to a gentle simmer.
3. Simmer for 3 hours, adding water as needed to keep the cans submerged.
4. Cool cans before opening. The sweetened, condensed milk becomes a rich, creamy, caramel-colored sauce, with a smooth consistency.
5. Transfer into a fondue pot to keep warm and serve with assorted dippers.

Chapter 14: Jack and Jill Showers for Couples: Diapers Wild!

Italian Sub Sandwiches
Serves 30

6-foot-long sub bun
3 pounds deli ham
3 pounds deli turkey or roast beef
2 pounds sliced salami
2 pounds provolone cheese
3 cups shredded lettuce
10 tomatoes, sliced
1 cup sliced hot banana peppers (optional)
½ cup bottled Italian dressing
Mayonnaise and mustard as desired

1. Slice the sub bun lengthwise, but not all the way through. Open it up flat like a book
2. Cover the bread with the slices of ham. Lay the turkey or beef on the ham, then the salami slices. Line up the cheese on top of the salami. Layer the lettuce, tomato, and banana peppers on the meats and cheese.
3. Drizzle dressing on the lettuce, and fold the sandwich closed.
4. Cut sandwich into thirty pieces with a serrated knife. Arrange on platter and serve.

Potato Salad with Egg
Serves 20

20 medium or 18 large potatoes

Cold water to cover with 2 tablespoons salt added

1½ cups cider vinegar

1½ cups mayonnaise

3 tablespoons dark honey mustard

10-ounce jar sweet gherkin pickles, chopped

12 hard-boiled eggs, peeled and chopped

1½ cups sweet onion, peeled and chopped

2 cups celery, rinsed and chopped

3 teaspoons celery salt or to taste

1. Peel the potatoes and cut into chunks. Put them in cold, salted water; bring to a boil. Boil potatoes until tender, about 20 minutes, depending on size. While the potatoes are cooking, prepare a large bowl for the salad by chilling it well.
2. Drain the potatoes, put them in the chilled bowl, and sprinkle them with the cider vinegar while they are still hot.
3. In a separate bowl, mix the rest of the ingredients together until very well combined to make the dressing.
4. Add the bowl of dressing and vegetables to the potatoes and mix to coat. Refrigerate until ready to serve.

Ice-Cream Sandwiches

For each sandwich you will need two 3" cookies and one scoop of your favorite ice cream. Cookies such as gingersnaps, chocolate chip, oatmeal raisin, and peanut butter make good homemade ice-cream sandwiches. To make the sandwiches, simply put a scoop of ice cream on one cookie, press another on top of the ice cream, and roll the sides in crushed cookie crumbs, nuts, or mini chocolate chips.

Chapter 14: Jack and Jill Showers for Couples: Lucky Strike!

Gutter-Ball Subs
Serves 8

32 (2") meatballs (store bought or from your favorite recipe)
3 cups marinara sauce
8 (6") sub buns
16 slices provolone cheese
2 cups shredded mozzarella cheese

1. Heat the meatballs in the sauce.
2. Open the buns flat and line them with provolone cheese.
3. Put 4 meatballs with sauce on each sandwich.
4. Sprinkle mozzarella cheese on top of meatballs.
5. Heat sandwiches in the oven at 350°F until cheese melts.

Kingpin Coleslaw
Serves 8

3 cups shredded cabbage
¼ cup shredded purple cabbage
¼ cup shredded carrot
¼ cup whole green onion, chopped
½ cup mayonnaise
1 tablespoon milk
1 teaspoon sugar
1 tablespoon cider vinegar
1 teaspoon celery seed
½ cup pumpkin seeds
Salt and pepper to taste

1. Mix all ingredients together.
2. Refrigerate at least 15 minutes before serving.

Hot Fudge Sauce
Makes 3 Cups

1 cup sugar
½ cup light corn syrup
1½ cups water
¾ cup cocoa powder
½ cup semisweet chocolate chips

1. In a saucepan over medium-high heat, stir together the sugar, corn syrup, and water. Bring to a boil. Boil for 5 minutes.
2. Stir the cocoa powder and chocolate chips into the sugar syrup until the chips are completely melted.
3. Remove from heat, strain, and refrigerate.

Butterscotch Sauce
Makes 1 Cup

1 cup dark brown sugar
⅓ cup heavy cream
4 tablespoons butter
2 tablespoons light corn syrup
1 teaspoon vanilla extract
1 tablespoon Scotch whiskey (optional)

1. Combine brown sugar, cream, butter, and corn syrup in a saucepan. Stir over low heat until sugar has dissolved.
2. Increase heat to medium, and simmer 5 minutes.
3. Remove from heat and stir in vanilla (and Scotch, if desired). Cool and store in the refrigerator for up to two weeks.

Chapter 14: Jack and Jill Showers for Couples: LaMaze–LeMans Car-Seat Rally

Trail Mix
Makes 8 Cups

> 2 cups raisins
> 2 cups dry-roasted peanuts
> 1 cup candy-coated chocolate (such as M&M's)
> 2 cups granola
> 1 cup shelled sunflower seeds

In a large bowl, combine all ingredients. Divide trail mix into individual portions and serve in paper cups or zippered plastic bags.

Chapter 15: Being Neighborly Showers: The Red Wagon Progressive Dinner

Limeade
Makes 12 Cups

> 1½ cups fresh-squeezed lime juice
> 8 cups water
> 1 cup sugar
> 1 cup lemon-lime soda
> Ice cubes

Combine lime juice, water, and sugar; add lemon-lime soda. Serve over ice.

Blue Corn Chips and Chunky Guacamole
Serves 8

2 large, ripe avocados
1 medium-sized red tomato
1 small yellow onion
½ cup canned jalapeño peppers
1 tablespoon lime juice
1 teaspoon salt
½ teaspoon ground black pepper

1. Cut the avocados in half lengthwise and pry out the pits. Remove the peels and cut the avocados into 1" pieces. Mash with a fork.
2. Cut the tomato into ½" pieces. Remove the skin from the onion and cut into ¼" pieces. Drain off the liquid from the jalapeño peppers and cut the peppers into ¼" pieces.
3. Combine all the ingredients; mix well.

Shrimp Crab Dip
Serves 12

4 ounces cream cheese, softened
1 cup cooked shrimp, chopped or popcorn size
1 cup canned crabmeat, drained and squeezed dry
1 cup diced celery
2 tablespoons minced onion
2 tablespoons chopped fresh parsley
¼ cup mayonnaise
2 teaspoons fresh lemon juice
¼ teaspoon sugar
¼ teaspoon pepper
⅛ teaspoon salt
2 drops cayenne-pepper sauce

1. With a mixer, beat the cream cheese until soft and fluffy.
2. Add the rest of the ingredients and mix thoroughly.
3. Chill for at least 2 hours before serving.

Hummus
Yields 2 Cups

6 cloves garlic, peeled
½ teaspoon salt
1 (14-ounce) can garbanzo beans
⅓ cup tahini (sesame-seed paste)
2 tablespoons fresh lemon juice
2 tablespoons olive oil
½ teaspoon ground cumin (optional)

1. Purée garlic and salt in food processor or blender. Add garbanzo beans and purée to a paste.
2. Add the remaining ingredients and blend until smooth.
3. Serve finished dip in a bowl or spread out on a platter. Drizzle with more olive oil and serve with raw vegetables or warmed pita wedges.

Hot and Sweet Italian Sausage
Serves 8

8 Italian frying peppers (light green skin)
½ cup olive oil, more if needed
3 sweet onions, thinly sliced
4 Italian hot sausages (about ⅓ to ½ pound each)
4 Italian sweet sausages (about ⅓ to ½ pound each)
2 (8-ounce) jars marinara sauce
8 split hero rolls or 4 loaves Italian bread, split and cut in half

1. Rinse and seed peppers, and cut into chunks.
2. Place olive oil in a pan over medium heat. Add peppers and sauté until they are soft. Add the onions and continue to sauté. (Add more olive oil if needed.) Once peppers and onions are cooked, remove from heat and set aside.
3. Place the sausages in boiling water for 10 minutes.
4. Preheat the grill to hot. Place the sauce in a pan to warm. Prepare the hero rolls or bread for toasting. Grill the sausages quickly, browning on each side. Toast bread while the sausages are grilling.
5. Build hero sandwiches on toasted bread: Add sausage and then peppers and onions. Top with marinara sauce, and put out plenty of paper napkins!

Spicy-Tart Apple Sauce
Makes 4 Cups

12 large, tart apples such as Granny Smith or Macintosh
Juice of 2 lemons and a 1" to 2" strip of lemon peel
1 cup water
4 tablespoons brown sugar
2 teaspoons ground cinnamon
½ teaspoon ground nutmeg
2 teaspoons salt
2 teaspoons Tabasco sauce (optional)

Peel, core, and coarsely chop the apples into chunks. Place the apples in a saucepan with the rest of the ingredients. Bring to a boil and then lower the heat. Simmer for 10 minutes. Serve hot or cold.

"Baby" Red Potatoes
Serves 8

6 pounds small red potatoes
8 tablespoons butter
4 tablespoons Dijon mustard
½ cup sliced whole green onions
Salt and pepper to taste

1. Shave an inch-wide belt around the middle of each potato with a vegetable peeler.
2. Place potatoes in a large pot in enough cold water to cover. Boil potatoes for 15 minutes or until they can be pierced easily with the tip of a paring knife.
3. Drain potatoes and toss them with butter, mustard, and green onions. Season with salt and pepper.

Greek Salad

Serves 8

    1 teaspoon dried oregano

    ½ cup olive oil

    3 tablespoons red wine vinegar

    Salt and pepper to taste

    2 heads romaine lettuce, chopped

    2 large tomatoes, chopped

    ½ red onion, sliced

    ½ cup black olives

    1 cucumber, sliced

    8 ounces feta cheese, crumbled

1. Make the salad dressing by whisking together oregano, oil, and vinegar. Season with salt and pepper.
2. Toss lettuce with dressing and put in a serving bowl.
3. Scatter vegetables and cheese over the dressed lettuce.

Strawberry Shortcake

Serves 8

Shortcake Dough:

    3 cups all-purpose flour

    4½ teaspoons baking powder

    1½ teaspoons salt

    1 tablespoon sugar

    6 tablespoons cold butter

    1¼ cups buttermilk

Strawberry Filling:

    Sugar for sprinkling

    4 cups (1 quart) whole strawberries

    1½ cups sugar

    3½ cups heavy cream

    1 teaspoon vanilla extract

    Powdered sugar

    8 sprigs mint (optional)

1. Preheat oven to 400°F.
2. Combine flour, baking powder, salt, and sugar in a mixing bowl.
3. Cut butter into small pieces and add to dry ingredients. Mix butter into dry ingredients with a pastry cutter or with your fingers. This mixture should be a bit lumpy so biscuits turn out flaky.
4. Add buttermilk and mix with a wooden spoon to form the dough.
5. Roll dough on a floured board to 1" thickness. Cut dough into circles with a 2" to 3" round cookie cutter or a drinking glass. Before baking, brush the

biscuits with some of the cream and sprinkle them with sugar. Place rounds on an ungreased baking sheet and bake 12 minutes.

6. When the biscuits are cool, split them horizontally and set aside.

7. Hull and slice the strawberries and toss them in a bowl with 1 cup of the sugar. Gently mash some of the berries with your hands. Set aside.

8. In a bowl, whip remaining cream (2 cups), ½ cup sugar, and vanilla to soft peaks, using an electric mixer or a whisk.

9. Assemble the shortcakes by placing one biscuit bottom on each plate. Top each biscuit bottom with a serving of strawberries. Put a dollop of whipped cream on top of the strawberries, and then top with the other biscuit half.

10. Garnish with a dusting of powdered sugar and a mint sprig.

Chapter 16: Showers for Dads: Extreme Nursery Makeover

Classic Reuben Sandwich
Serves 4

> 1 cup sauerkraut, very well drained
> 2 tablespoons unsalted butter, divided
> 8 slices rye bread
> ⅓ cup Thousand Island or Russian dressing
> ½ pound Swiss cheese, thinly sliced
> ½ pound corned beef, thinly sliced

1. Be sure the sauerkraut is well drained, using a paper towel if necessary. Heat 1 tablespoon of the butter in a large skillet over medium to medium-high heat. While butter is melting, spread one side of 4 pieces of bread with dressing. Lay the bread, dressing-side up, in the skillet, moving the bread around to fully coat with butter. Layer the cheese, sauerkraut, and corned beef on the bread in the skillet.

2. With the remaining bread slices, butter one side and spread the other with dressing. Top the sandwiches in the skillet, placing the bread butter-side up. Press down firmly. After the sandwiches have cooked for about 5 minutes on one side, carefully flip with a spatula. Press down firmly again. Cover the skillet for about 3 to 4 minutes, or until the cheese has melted and the second side is golden. Serve hot with kosher dill pickles, if desired.

Macaroni Salad
Serves 6–8

4 cups cooked macaroni
½ cup thinly sliced celery
1 tablespoon minced pimiento
1 cup mayonnaise
¼ cup sliced green olives
2 tablespoons chopped fresh parsley
Salt and pepper to taste
4 eggs
Paprika

1. Place eggs in a saucepan with cold water that rises about an inch above the eggs. Bring the water to a boil and cover the saucepan. Boil eggs for 20 minutes, then run under cold water. Remove shells and thinly slice eggs.
2. Mix all ingredients except eggs and paprika in a bowl. Chill for 1 hour.
3. Cover the surface with sliced eggs, sprinkle with paprika, and serve.

Cake-Mix Cookies
Yields 36-40 Cookies

1 package yellow cake mix
¼ cup vegetable oil
2 teaspoons water
2 eggs
1 cup semisweet chocolate morsels
1 cup nuts, chopped

1. Preheat oven to 375°F.
2. In a large bowl, mix together all the ingredients to form a soft dough. Using your hands, form the dough into small balls the size of walnuts. Place on ungreased baking sheets, spacing the balls about 2" apart.
3. Bake for 10–12 minutes, or until delicately browned. Let cool on the baking sheets for a few minutes before removing to racks to cool completely.

Baby-Back Barbeque Short Ribs
Serves 8

8 cloves garlic, unpeeled
8–10 pounds meaty, short ribs of beef
1 cup cider vinegar
2 cups apple cider
4 onions, unpeeled and quartered
4 tablespoons red-pepper flakes
4 tablespoons juniper berries, bruised in a mortar and pestle
Apple-wood briquettes and 2 cups presoaked apple-wood chips
3 cups Spicy Barbecue Sauce (page 264)

1. Smash the garlic cloves under a wide blade or frying pan. In a large container, cover the short ribs with water and add the vinegar, cider, onions, garlic, and spices. Soak, refrigerated, overnight.
2. In a large pot with a cover, add enough water to the marinade to cover the ribs. Simmer on stove for 2 hours.
3. Prepare the grill with the wood chips and briquettes.
4. Grill or smoke the ribs over barbecue about 1 hour, or until brown and juicy, brushing often with sauce. When glossy brown but not burned, serve on a platter.

Spicy Barbeque Sauce
Makes 1 Quart

½ cup olive oil

2 onions, peeled and chopped

4–5 cloves garlic, peeled and chopped

4 jalapeño peppers, cored, de-ribbed, seeded, and chopped

2 canned chipotle peppers, chopped

1 red Scotch bonnet pepper, cored, seeded, and chopped

1 quart fresh or canned tomatoes

2 cups chili sauce

1 teaspoon ground cloves

½ teaspoon ground cinnamon

2 bay leaves

2 tablespoons dark brown sugar

½ cup cider vinegar

2 teaspoons salt

1 tablespoon prepared brown mustard

1 ounce bittersweet chocolate

1 tablespoon liquid smoke (optional)

¼ cup bourbon, rum, or tequila (optional)

1. Heat the oil in a large soup kettle. Add the onions, garlic, three kinds of peppers, and tomatoes. Sauté until soft.
2. Add the rest of the ingredients and stir. Cover and simmer for 2 hours, reducing to 1 quart.
3. Remove bay leaves and whirl in blender until smooth. Cool and place in a jar. This will keep for at least a week.

Chuck-Wagon Kidney Beans
Serves 6–8

½ cup olive oil
1 red onion, chopped
4 cloves garlic, minced
1 sweet red pepper, cored, seeded, and chopped
2 serrano chilies, or to taste, cored, seeded, and minced
2 Scotch bonnet chilies, or to taste, cored, seeded, and minced
1 pound dried kidney beans in water to cover, soaked overnight
1 pound ground beef
1 (29-ounce) can crushed tomatoes
1 can low-salt beef broth
1 tablespoon instant coffee dissolved in ¼ cup hot water
2 tablespoons cocoa powder dissolved in ¼ cup cold water
1 bottle beer (not dark or light, use regular)
1 tablespoon Worcestershire sauce
1 teaspoon ground cinnamon
1 teaspoon ground cumin
1 teaspoon dried thyme
2 tablespoons chili powder
½ cup red wine
Salt and freshly ground black pepper to taste

1. Heat the olive oil in a large, heavy-bottomed soup pot. Add the onion, garlic, and peppers; sauté over low heat, stirring for 5 minutes.
2. Blend in the rest of the ingredients, cover, and simmer for 5–6 hours.
3. Serve in bowls garnished with sour cream, chopped scallions, and grated Cheddar cheese. A bowl of taco chips on the side is a classic accompaniment.

Beefsteak Tomatoes and Onions with Italian-Dressing Marinade
Serves 8

8 beefsteak tomatoes, in thick slices
4 red onions, sliced thin
1 bottle of Italian-style salad dressing—your choice

1. Put tomatoes and onions in a sealable plastic container.
2. Drizzle with dressing and toss until well coated.
3. Let marinate for several hours in the refrigerator. Serve with ribs.

Chuck-Wagon Cornbread
Makes 8 Pieces

4 slices bacon, fried and drained on paper towel, fat reserved
2–4 jalapeño peppers, cored, seeded, and minced
4 scallions, chopped
1 tablespoon butter
¾ cup yellow or white cornmeal
1½ cups all-purpose flour
2 teaspoons double-action baking powder
½ teaspoon salt
1 cup buttermilk
2 tablespoons molasses or brown sugar
2 whole eggs

1. Fry the bacon, then drain and reserve the fat. After the bacon has been removed from the pan, sauté the peppers and scallions in the reserved fat, adding a tablespoon of butter if the pan gets dry. Remove from the heat. Crumble the bacon and mix it with the peppers and scallions.
2. Measure the cornmeal, flour, baking powder, and salt into the bowl of an electric mixer. With the motor on low, blend in the buttermilk. Then add the rest of the ingredients, scraping the bowl from time to time.
3. Preheat the oven to 400°F. Prepare an 8"-square pan with nonstick spray.
4. Pour half of the batter into the pan. Spread with the bacon, pepper, and scallion mixture. Pour the rest of the batter on top.
5. Bake for about 25 minutes or until golden brown.

Cheesecake
Serves 12

½ cup all-purpose flour
2 tablespoons sugar
6 tablespoons butter, melted
½ cup ground almonds
24 ounces cream cheese (do not use whipped cream cheese), softened
2 cups sugar
2 tablespoons cornstarch
3 eggs
3½ cups sour cream
1 teaspoon vanilla extract

1. Preheat oven to 350°F. In a bowl, combine flour, 2 tablespoons sugar, melted butter, and ground almonds with a rubber spatula. Press mixture into the bottom of a springform pan that has been sprayed with cooking spray. Bake for 10 minutes. Remove from oven and set aside.
2. With an electric mixer, beat the cream cheese until fluffy. Add 1½ cups of the sugar and the cornstarch; cream together. Beat in eggs one at a time, scraping down the sides of the bowl after each one. Stir in 1½ cups of the sour cream.
3. Pour this batter into the springform pan and bake for about 1 hour. The middle of the cheesecake should jiggle slightly when finished. Remove from oven and cool at room temperature. Refrigerate and chill completely overnight.
4. With an electric mixer, whip 2 cups of sour cream with ½ cup sugar and the vanilla.
5. Top the chilled cheesecake with the whipped sour cream mixture; smooth the top. Let the cake set in the refrigerator, covered, for 1–2 hours before serving.

Chapter 18: e-Showers: The Desktop Shower: Coffee-Break Contractions

Fresh Scones
Makes 16

3 cups all-purpose flour
6 tablespoons sugar, plus more for sprinkling
1 teaspoon salt
3 teaspoons baking powder
12 tablespoons cold, unsalted butter, cut in pieces
4 eggs
⅓ cup heavy cream
1 teaspoon vanilla extract

1. Preheat oven to 400°F. Line a cookie sheet with parchment paper, or brush lightly with oil. (You could alternately spray the cookie sheet with cooking spray.)
2. Combine flour, sugar, salt, baking powder, and butter in a food processor with a metal blade, or use two butter knives to mix dry ingredients while chopping up butter into smaller pieces. Cut butter until mixture resembles cornmeal.
3. In a large bowl combine eggs, cream, and vanilla using a whisk.
4. Fold in dry ingredients with a spatula. Drop scones into rounds onto prepared cookie sheet.
5. Sprinkle scones with sugar and bake for 15 minutes.

Biscotti
Makes 20

4 tablespoons unsalted butter, softened
¼ cup sugar
1 egg
½ teaspoon vanilla extract
1 teaspoon baking powder
Pinch of salt
1 cup all-purpose flour
½ cup whole almonds

1. Preheat oven to 350°F. Lay the almonds out in an even layer on an ungreased baking sheet pan; bake for 10 minutes. Set aside. Keep the oven on for the biscotti.
2. Grease a baking sheet.
3. Cream the butter, egg, and sugar together with the salt and flour. Add this dry mixture to the egg/butter mixture, and combine to make a smooth dough. Stir in almonds.
4. Scrape dough out onto the prepared baking sheet. Wet your fingers with water, and then form the dough into a broad, flat log. Bake for 30 minutes at 350°F. Remove from the oven and cool on the baking sheet for 5 minutes. Turn down the oven to 275°F.
5. Remove the log to a cutting board. Cut the log into ½"-wide slices and place the slices back on the baking sheet, cut sides facing up. Bake 15 minutes; turn cookies over and bake 10 minutes more. Remove from pan and cool on a rack.

Coffee Cake
Serves 12–16

½ cup dark brown sugar
2 teaspoons cinnamon
3½ cups all-purpose flour
1 cup cold butter
1½ cups sugar
3 eggs
2 teaspoons baking powder
1 teaspoon baking soda
½ teaspoon salt
1 cup sour cream

1. Preheat oven to 350°F. Butter a Bundt pan.
2. Make filling by combining the brown sugar, cinnamon, ⅓ cup of the flour, and ¼ cup of the butter with fingertips until crumbly. Set aside.
3. For the batter: Cream together ¾ cup butter and sugar until fluffy. Add eggs one at a time and beat them to form a smooth batter. Separately, mix together 3 cups flour, baking powder, baking soda, and salt, using a whisk.

4. Add flour mixture alternately with sour cream to the butter/egg mixture until all is incorporated. Layer half the batter in the Bundt pan; sprinkle it with the filling mixture. Layer the rest of the batter on top.

5. Bake 50 minutes, or until a toothpick inserted in the middle comes out clean. Sprinkle with powdered sugar before serving in slices.

Chocolate Yummies
Makes 12 Squares

1½ cups (18 squares) graham-cracker crumbs
12-ounce can sweetened condensed milk
6-ounce package semisweet chocolate morsels

1. Preheat oven to 350°F. Butter an 8"-square cake pan.
2. Place the crumbs in the prepared pan and add the milk. Mix until the crumbs are moist. Add the chocolate morsels. Spread evenly in the pan. Bake for 30 minutes, or until firm. Remove from the oven; let cool.
3. Variation: If you want, add ½ cup chopped nuts with the chocolate chips.

Chapter 18: e-Showers: The "Lap-Top" Shower Visit

Tortilla Lasagna
Serves 8

½ cup chopped onion	¼ teaspoon cumin
1 clove garlic, minced	3 cups enchilada sauce
1 teaspoon olive oil	12 corn tortillas
1 pound ground turkey	2 cups shredded Monterey Jack cheese

1. Preheat oven to 400°F. Sauté onions and garlic in oil. Add turkey and cook until it is browned. Stir in cumin. Set aside.
2. Spoon a layer of enchilada sauce on the bottom of a 9" × 13" casserole dish. Layer tortillas, meat mixture, and cheese; then sauce, tortillas, meat, and cheese again. Top with a layer of tortillas, sauce, and cheese.
3. Bake 15–20 minutes.

Chicken with Rice
Serves 6

3 boneless, skinless chicken breasts, cubed
½ cup olive oil
1 large onion, diced
1 cup diced green bell pepper
½ cup diced red bell pepper
½ cup diced yellow bell pepper
5 cloves garlic, minced
1 tablespoon turmeric
3 cups white long-grain rice, uncooked
4 cups chicken broth
¾ cup chopped green olives
2 bay leaves
Salt and pepper to taste

1. Brown chicken in oil in a large pot. Remove chicken and set aside.
2. Add onion, peppers, garlic, and turmeric to the pot, and sauté until onions are translucent.
3. Add rice and cook for 5 minutes, stirring occasionally. Add chicken broth, browned chicken, olives, and bay leaves. Stir to combine, bring mixture to a simmer over medium heat, and cover pot with a lid.
4. Simmer 20 minutes or until rice is cooked.
5. Remove bay leaves. Season with salt and pepper.

Quickie Pasta Bake
Serves 6

1 tablespoon olive oil
1 onion, chopped
2 cloves garlic, minced
1 (28-ounce) can tomatoes, crushed
1 teaspoon oregano
Salt and pepper to taste
1 pound ziti or rotini, cooked and drained
2 cups grated cheese, any type

1. Preheat the oven to 350°F. Heat the oil in a heavy, large, ovenproof skillet. Add the onion and garlic; sauté till soft (about 5 minutes). Add the tomatoes, oregano, salt, and pepper. Cook till heated through, about 5 minutes. Add the cooked pasta and ½ cup grated cheese to the mixture. Sprinkle the remaining cheese on the top.
2. Bake 15 to 20 minutes or until cheese on top is bubbly.

Oven-Fried Chicken Nuggets
Serves 4

8 tablespoons butter, melted

2 tablespoons Dijon mustard

3 cups dry breadcrumbs

1 cup Parmesan cheese

1 tablespoon onion powder

2 teaspoons paprika

2 teaspoons salt

1 teaspoon pepper

3 boneless, skinless chicken breasts,
    cut in chunks

1. Preheat oven to 350°F. Line a baking sheet with foil and set aside.
2. Melt butter and mix it with the mustard. Set aside.
3. Combine bread crumbs, Parmesan cheese, onion powder, paprika, salt, and pepper in a bowl. Set aside.
4. Toss chicken chunks in the butter mixture; then roll them around in the crumb mixture.
5. Arrange the coated chicken chunks on the foil and bake for 1 hour. Serve warm or at room temperature.

Real Macaroni and Cheese
Serves 6

4 tablespoons butter

¼ cup all-purpose flour

1 teaspoon dry mustard

2¾ cups milk

1 teaspoon salt

⅛ teaspoon pepper

Pinch cayenne pepper

3 cups shredded Cheddar cheese

16 ounces elbow macaroni, cooked and drained

1 cup dry bread crumbs

1. Preheat oven to 350°F. Butter a 9" × 13" baking dish.
2. Melt the butter in a medium-size saucepan. Stir in the flour and dry mustard; cook (stirring) over medium heat for 2 minutes.
3. Add the milk and whisk over medium heat until mixture thickens, whisking constantly to prevent burning on the bottom. Stir in the salt, pepper, and cayenne pepper. Remove from heat.
4. Stir in the cheese and let the mixture sit for a minute. Stir again to smooth out the melted cheese.
5. Pour cooked macaroni into the casserole dish; add cheese sauce. Mix until macaroni is coated with cheese.
6. Sprinkle bread crumbs on top of the casserole and bake for 45 minutes, until browned and bubbly on the edges. Serve warm.

Black-Bottom Cupcakes
Makes 12

8 ounces cream cheese, softened	½ cup cocoa powder
⅓ cup sugar	2 teaspoons baking soda
1 egg	1 teaspoon salt
Pinch of salt	2 cups cold water
1 cup semisweet chocolate chips	⅔ cup vegetable oil
3 cups all-purpose flour	2 tablespoons distilled vinegar
2 cups sugar	2 teaspoons vanilla extract

1. Make the filling by combining the cream cheese, ⅓ cup sugar, egg, pinch of salt, and chocolate chips. Refrigerate until ready to use. (Can be made up to three days in advance.)
2. Preheat oven to 325°F. Put twelve fluted paper cups in a muffin tin and set aside.
3. Combine the flour, 2 cups sugar, cocoa powder, baking soda, and salt in a mixing bowl.
4. In a pitcher, combine the water, oil, and vanilla. Pour the wet ingredients into the dry ingredients and whip with an electric mixer for 3 minutes. Pour the batter evenly into the prepared muffin tin. Top each cupcake with 1–2 tablespoons of the cream-cheese filling.
5. Bake for 28 minutes. Cool in the pan before serving.

Appendix A

Resources

Activities

Art Gallery Tour
212-946-1548
www.nygallerytours.com/private.htm

Food Tours
Foods of New York Tours, Inc.
Call 212-802-7197 to make reservations
http://foodsofny.com

Zen Zoo Tea Cafe
310-860-0688
www.zenzootea.com

Baby Gear

Bling Baby Pacifier, Etc.
Paci Posh LLC
www.shopbabyposh.com

Bowling Bunnies
Genius Babies, Inc.
2015 Van Buren Avenue
Indian Trail, NC 28079
704-893-2113
http://geniusbabies.com/chilsofbowpl.html

Diaper Daddy's Tool Belt
Baby Shower Depot
P.O. Box 10475
New Brunswick, NJ 08906-0475
732-287-4195
info@babyshowerdepot.com
http://babyshowerdepot.com/daddy-baby-shower-gifts.html

Frog Pod Bath Toy Storage
Boon Inc.
5005 S. Ash Avenue, Suite A-18
Tempe, AZ 85282
888-376-4763
Fax: 480-718-8833
www.booninc.com

Nursing Chair with Lumbar Support
Monarch Nursery
1-866-786-6222
www.monarchnursery.com

Nursery Equipment Safety Checklist
health.yahoo.com/media/healthwise/form_ue5205.pdf

**Sleep Sheep from Cloud b and L'ovedbaby
4-in-1 Nursing Shawl**
Bare Babies
17815 Newhope Street, Suite F
Fountain Valley, CA 92708
1-800-220-7743
✍*www.barebabies.com*

Stay-Put Sunglasses
6032 N. 31st Street
Phoenix, AZ 85016
1-888-MY-FRUBI
Fax: 1-877-GO-FRUBI
✍*www.frubishades.com*

Swaddling Star
10517 NE 46th Street
Kirkland, WA 98033
206-284-3404 or 800-518-3339
Fax: 206-284-7828

Under Construction Bookends
Nova Lighting
P.O. Box 58327
Los Angeles, CA 90058
323-277-6266
Fax: 323-277-6270
✍*www.novalamps.com*

Skin Products for Babies

Boots Gentle Skin Care Products
Boots Retail USA Inc.
177 Broad Street, Suite 1050
Stamford, CT 06901
1-866-75-BOOTS
✍*www.boots.com*

Burt's Bees Inc.
P.O. Box 13489
Durham, NC 27709
866-422-8787
✍*www.burtsbees.com*

Natural Organic Skin Care Products
Earth Mama Angel Baby
9866 SE Empire Court
Clackamas, OR 97015
503-607-0607
Fax: 503-607-0667
✍*www.earthmamaangelbaby.com*

Mustela
Expanscience Laboratories dba Mustela
1537 Waukegan Road
Waukegan, IL 60085
1-800-422-2987
✍*www.mustela.com*

Clothing

Aprons
AllHeartChefs.com—Professional Appearances, Inc.
5284 Adolfo Road, Suite 250
Camarillo, CA 93012
1-805-384-4425
Fax: 1-805-445-8816
✍*www.allheartchefs.com/solidaprons.html*

Baby Bowler T-Shirts
Lingo T-shirts
1-877-809-1659
www.lingotshirts.com/bowling.htm

Baby Bunches
1-877-456-2229
✍*www.thebabybunch.com/#/apparel*

Cheeritoes
Genius Babies, Inc.
2015 Van Buren Avenue
Indian Trail, NC 28079
704-893-2113
*http://geniusbabies.com/cheeritoes-box
-of-baby-socks.html*

Due Maternity
1-866-SHOP-DUE
www.duematernity.com

iMaternity
1-800-466-6223
www.imaternity.com

Mom's the Word
1-877-452-6667
www.momsthewordmaternity.com

Maternity Exchange
www.maternityxchange.com

Mercedes Hill Maternity
2440 Emmons Ave
Rochester Hills, MI 48307
888-868-8095
www.mercedeshill.com

Pickles and Ice Cream
5001 Spring Valley Road, Suite 385-W
Dallas, TX 75244
1-888-4-9-MONTHS (888-496-6684) or
214-PICKLES (214-742-5537)
www.picklesandicecream.com

Theatre Baby Onesie
*www.cafepress.com/buy/theatre%20onesie/-/
cfpt2_/cfpt_source_searchBox/copt_*

Customized Gifts

Baby Hats and Custom Baseball Glove
1-800-671-0886
www.annabean.com

Art Cabinets
Dynamic Frames Inc.
310-320-6302 or 1-800-579-7191
Fax: 310-320-6289
www.dynamicframes.com/artframes.htm

Belly Casting Kit
Doula Shop
www.doulashop.com

Belly Gifts
*www.bellygifts.com/Proud-Body-Belly-Casting
-Kit-p/182.htm*

Crossword Puzzles
http://pdos.csail.mit.edu/cgi-bin/theme-cword
www.personalpuzzles.com
www.varietygames.com

Custom Children's Books
I See Me! Inc.
1101 Fourth Street North
Cannon Falls, MN 55009
1-877-281-0536
www.iseeme.com

Custom Lunch Boxes
WaDaYaNeed, LLC
P.O. Box 296, 1516-1 State Route 7
Warnerville, NY 12187
1-800-958-4332
Fax: 518 234-8593
*www.wadayaneed.com/largeplasticlunch
boxescustomimprintedpromotionallogo.htm*

Custom Mouse Pads
2617 Karluk Street
Anchorage, AK 99508
1-866-404-5267
Fax: 907-569-1702
www.custommousepad.com/pricing.html

DNA Art
70 George Street, Suite 200
Ottawa, Ontario K1N 5V9 Canada
1-866-619-9574
www.dna11.com

Personalized Wine Labels
Personal Wine
512-476-WINE (9463) or 1-800-690-WINE (9463)
www.personalwine.com

Photo Album
Ronnie Gousman
Bookbinding
Los Angeles, CA
323-651-2900

Presidential Greeting for Newborn Babies
White House Greetings, Washington, DC 20500
Include: Name of new baby, address informa-
tion, and date of birth

Name a Star
International Star Registry
34523 Wilson Road
Ingleside, IL 60041
1-800-282-3333
www.starregistry.com

Dad's Shower

Eco-Friendly Paint
*http://eartheasy.com/live_nontoxic_paints
.htm#2d*

Anna Sova
2263 Valdina Street
Dallas, Texas 75207
1-877-326-7682
Fax: 214-744-0830
www.annasova.com

Geochaching
Groundspeak, Inc.
PMB 321
24 Roy Street
Seattle, WA 98109
206-302-7721
www.geocaching.com/faq

Real Milk Paint
11 West Pumping Station Road
Quakertown, PA 18951
1-800-339-9748
Fax: 215-538-5435
www.realmilkpaint.com

Décor

Aprons
AllHeartChefs.com—Professional Appearances,
Inc.
5284 Adolfo Road, Suite 250
Camarillo, CA 93012
805-384-4425
Fax: 805-445-8816
www.allheartchefs.com/solidaprons.html

Diaper Cake

Lil Baby Cakes
DWP LLC
P.O. Box 1414
Huntersville, NC 28070
1-866-944-2253
✆www.lilbabycakes.com

Luminarias

LumaBase
610-524-4166
✆www.lumabase.com

Mini Red Wagon

Radio Flyer Inc.
6515 West Grand Avenue
Chicago, Illinois 60707
1-800-621-7613
✆www.radioflyer.com/accessories/minis_
accessories.html

Wire-Sculptured Baby Carriage

Plum Party
30-00 47th Avenue
Long Island City, NY 11101
718-433-2484 or 1-800-227-0314
✆www.plumparty.com

Red Carpet Rental

Grand Carpets
P.O. Box 22
Bath, PA 18014-0022
1-877-594-7166
✆www.grandcarpets.com

Favors

Bath Salts Tea

Victoria's Soaps & Scents
11730 Cape Cod Lane
Huntley, IL 60142
1-847-275-1067
Fax: 509-461-3073
✆www.victoriasoapsandscents.com/64.html

Candy Pacifiers (Popcifiers)

Blair Candy
1215 7th Avenue
Altoona, PA 16602
1-800-698-3536
Fax: 814-944-8470
✆www.blaircandy.com/glopapolo12.html

Chef Hats

KNG International
2102 East Karcher Road
Nampa, ID 83687
1-800-888-MENU (6368)
✆www.kng.com

Felt Bags

Plum Party
30-00 47th Avenue
Long Island City, NY 11101
718-433-2484 or 1-800-227-0314
✆www.plumparty.com/page/100200/CTGY/
groovyholidaysalloccasions

Flower Flip Flops

Oriental Trading Company, Inc.
1-800-875-8480
✆www.orientaltrading.com

Little I Lipstick Mint Mirror

My Wedding Favors
3012 Adriatic Court
Norcross, GA 30071
1-866-942-1311
www.myweddingfavors.com/mirror-mints.html

Lollipop Pots

Michaels and Kendon Candies
460 Perrymont Avenue
San Jose, CA 95125
1-800-33-CANDY
Fax: 408-297-4008
www.kendoncandies.com

Mug Holders

2850 Ocean Park Boulevard, Suite 310
Santa Monica, CA 90405
1-877-999-2433
www.cooking.com

Pink Polka-Dot Manicure Purses

Simply Baby Stuff
1921 Talen Street
Menomonie, WI 54751
1-800-274-4282
www.simplybabystuff.com/ppopumaset.html

Shoe Favors

DBC Collectibles
950 Ridge Road
Unit A13
Claymont, DE 19703
1-800-416-0690
*www.dbccollectibles.com/right_shoe/shoe.
    php?gclid=CPOVMqup4sCFR0dYAodNV5EfQ*

Food

Barbequed Ribs

www.corkysbbq.com/store.htm
www.jackstackbbq.com

Bakery Goods

Gianna's Grille
507 South 6th Street
Philadelphia, PA 19147-1408
215-829-GG4U
www.giannasgrille.com/bakery_order.html

Bubblegum Cigars and Kiss Labels

National Events Group, Ltd
8654 Cotter Street
Lewis Center, OH 43035
1-866-290-3615
www.abcfavors.com

Bubble Tea Pearls

Bubble Tea Supply
1466 Liliha Street
Honolulu, HI 96817
1-808-948-BOBA (2622)
*www.bubbleteasupply.com/index
    .php?page=recipes.html*

Chocolate Instruments

Chocolate Vault
8475 Chicago Road (US 12)
Horton, MI 79246
1-517-688-3388 or 1-800-525-1165
www.chocolatevault.com/music.htm

Coffee Packets Customized

The Chocolate Candy Roses Co.
P.O. Box 502586
San Diego, CA 92150-2586
760-751-8690
*www.sayitwithfavors.com/DDBaby
Cappuccino.html*

Chocolate Pump and Purse

Sweet Bliss
212-842-2773
www.sweetbliss.com

Food Preparation System

KidCo, Inc.
1013 Technology Way
Libertyville, IL 60048
847-549-8600 or 1-800-553-5529
Fax: 847-549-8660
www.kidco.com

Frozen Hot Chocolate

Serendipity 3
225 East 60th Street
New York, NY 10022
212-838-3531
www.serendipity3.com/main.htm

Lobster Bake

1-800-360-9520
www.thelobsternet.com

Hard Apple Cider

Warwick Valley Winery
P.O. Box 354
Warwick, New York 10990
845-258-4858
www.wvwinery.com/cider_02.html

Imported Foods

P.O. Box 2054
Issaquah, WA 98027
1-888-618-THAI (8424)
http://importfood.com/bubbletea.html

Mini Chocolate Champagne Bottles

CandyWarehouse.com, Inc.
5314 Third Street
Irwindale, CA 91706-2060
626-480-0899
*www.candywarehouse.com/mini
champagne.html*

Organic Baby Food

Homemade Baby
10335 W. Jefferson Boulevard
Culver City, CA 90232
1-800-854-8507
www.homemadebaby.com

Torani Syrup

Lollicup USA, Inc. Corporate Office
1100 Coiner Court
City of Industry, CA 91748
626-965-8882
Fax: 626-965-8729
www.lollicupstore.com/toranisyrups.html

World Wide Chocolates

P.O. Box 77
Center Strafford, NH 03815
1-800-664-9410
*www.worldwidechocolate.com/shop_
domori.html*

Invitations

Academy Awards Ticket Invitation
Kamyra in Print
886 Marimba Drive
El Paso, TX 79912
✍*www.partyinvitations.com/order/order_
    ticket_academy_awards.htm*

Blue Print Invitation
Write Expressions Studio
Wake Forest, North Carolina
919-562-4136
Fax: 775-582-4136
✍*www.writeexpressionsstudio.com/store/
    Details.cfm?ProdID=659&category=7*

Film Canister for Invitation
Plum Party
30-00 47th Avenue
Long Island City, NY 11101
718-433-2484 or 1-800-227-0314
✍*www.plumparty.com/partysupplies/17666.html*

Paper Dolls
Marilee's Paperdolls
✍*http://marilee.us/paperdolls3.html#Printadults*

Red Wagon Invitations
Party Pail, Inc.
718 Griffin Avenue, #338
Enumclaw, WA 98022

Shoe Invitations
Plum Party
30-00 47th Avenue
Long Island City, NY 11101
718-433-2484 or 1-800-227-0314
✍*www.plumparty.com/partysupplies/19591.html*

The Stationery Studio
847-541-5800
Fax: 847-5850
✍*www.thestationerystudio.com*

Tiny Prints
201 San Antonio Circle, Suite 235
Mountain View, CA 94040
1-877-300-9256
Fax: 650-249-3578
✍*www.tinyprints.com/baby_shower.htm*

Ticket Shower Invites and Save-the-Dates
Special Event Ticketing
20 Imperial Circle
Saint Charles, MO 63303
314-787-8107
✍*www.specialeventticketing.
    com/site/790667/page/906823*

Massage

Baby Massage
International Association of Infant Massage
Box 81
942 22 Älvsbyn
Sweden
Tel: (Sweden) 46 929 14236
Fax: (Sweden) 46 929 10747
✍*www.iaim.net*

Baby Yoga Fashions
Baby Yogi Gifts
2 John Wise Avenue
Essex, MA 01929
978-768-3112
✍*www.babyyogigifts.com/fashion.php*

Infant Massage Institute
605 Bledsoe Road NW
Albuquerque, NM 87107
505-341-9381
Fax: 505-341-9386
www.infantmassageinstitute.com

Infant Massage USA
7481 Huntsman Blvd, Suite 635
Springfield, VA 22153
703-455-3455 or 1-800-497-5996
www.infantmassageusa.org

Misc./General

Clear Labels
Computer Supplies
3069 McCall Drive, Suite 14
Atlanta, GA 30340
770-986-0135 or 1-800-419-2466
Fax: 770-986-6035
www.data-labels.com/clearlaslab.html?
gclid=CJjX3JDNnYwCFR1Bggodoh086Q

Poker Resources

Poker Cards
Cara Gail's
www.caragails.com

Poker Chip Make-Your-Own Labels
Online Labels, Inc.
925 Florida Central Parkway
Longwood, FL 32750
1-888-575-2235
Fax: 1-866-406-7341
www.onlinelabels.com/ol1025.htm

Poker Rules and Tournament Ideas
Home Poker Tourney
www.homepokertourney.com/rules_poker.htm

Poker Tournament Software
MB Hammond Group LLC
14428 Walton-Verona Road
Verona, KY 41092
www.pokertournamentmanager.com

United States Poker Association
www.foruspa.org/laws-of-poker.pdf

Teddy Bear Resources

Bear Stamps
Stamps By Impression
P.O. Box 641
Lewes, DE 19958
302-645-7191
www.stampsbyimpression.com/bears

Teddy Bear Kits
Ted E. Makers
1-888-55-TEDDY
http://erteestate.stores.yahoo.net/index.html

Appendix B

Project Directions

All project directions and illustrations are available online at *www.everydayeventplanner.com*.

Chapter 7: Painted Canvas "Baby Quilt"

This lovely painted quilt won't keep baby warm at night, but the love with which it was made will keep baby warm for years to come.

Materials Needed:

✓ Acrylic paint. 10 tubes in appointed colors plus 1 large tube of Burnt Umber for undercoating painting, black and white paint. TIP: Mixing paint to achieve consistent colors can be tricky. Try to buy colors that are close to the way you envision the "quilt" in your head to avoid the need to mix more paint.

✓ 8–12 10" to 12"-square wrap-around canvases that are 1" deep

✓ Assorted paint brushes of decent quality. ½" flat bristle brushes and a lettering brush for details

✓ Water containers to rinse brushes

✓ Muffin tin to mix and hold paints or plastic cups

✓ Newspaper to protect the work surfaces

Directions:

1. Before guests arrive you should prime canvases. To prime a canvas you simply brush it with a slightly thinned cup containing burnt sienna paint. It is not necessary to cover every inch of the canvas. Do this step one to two days prior to the shower.

2. Set up work stations. This is a great project for a backyard or patio if weather permits. Cover all work surfaces. Place brushes, water, and paints so that each person has access to them as they work.

3. Choose a design or narrow the options down. Pick something that the whole group can agree upon or that will go with the basic nursery decor. Have a copy of the basic design available for each person to work from. Have each person mark off the basics of the design in pencil over the prepainted canvas.

4. Start painting. Acrylic paints can be thinned with water, but they shouldn't be too runny. Encourage creativity within the basic design. Let each artist add their own squiggles and dots to make their canvas unique. Remember to have guests paint the outside edges of the canvas.

5. When the paintings are finished, place them in an area to dry completely. Finish by attaching a hook to the back of each one for hanging.

Chapter 10: Button Theme and Decor Ideas

The baby and button border designed for this party can be used in a variety of ways to create consistent and adorable party décor.

Materials Needed for a Border of Buttons on a Tablecloth or Runner:

✓ 1 white or light-colored cotton tablecloth or table runner in desired size

✓ 1 package of dark fabric T-shirt transfer paper

✓ 1 computer with scanner and color printer

✓ Scissors

✓ Heavy-duty iron

✓ Hard surface to use for ironing clothing. A regular metal ironing board is not recommended by manufacturer.

Directions:

1. Scan the design you wish to use into your computer. Make any adjustments you want to customize the look of your transfer design. When you are satisfied with the end product, print out onto specialty transfer paper. You should be able to get several images onto one transfer sheet. Save images as JPEG files.
2. Cut out around images and get ready to place.
3. Place the images where you want them on the cloth. Cover picture with the contact sheet that comes with the transfer paper.
4. Iron-on designs as instructed by transfer-paper manufacturer.

5. You may embellish the T-shirts with fabric paints or just leave them as they are.

Ideas for Button Placement:

✓ Run two rows of buttons around the edge of the table cloth.

✓ Create a grid of buttons over entire cloth.

✓ For a runner, create five rows of buttons across each end.

✓ Go for simplicity—run a single row of buttons down through the table center.

Chapter 10: Cute-as-a-Button Wall Hanging

NOTE: Get the wall hanging complete to the button-sewing stage before your party. Then let guests help sew on buttons. See *www .everydayeventplanner.com* for ideas and layout.

Materials Needed:

✓ 1 of Button A

✓ 2 of Button B

✓ 3 of Button C

✓ 4 of Button D

✓ 5 of Button E

✓ 6 of Button F

✓ 7 of Button G

✓ 8 of Button H

✓ 9 of Button I

✓ 10 of Button J

✓ 1 extra button from each guest

✓ ¾ yard fleece for front

- ✓ ¾ yard fleece in contrasting color for numbers and back
- ✓ 1 yard nonwoven interfacing
- ✓ 36" curtain rod with fanciful ends and brackets for hanging
- ✓ 2 packages (4 yards each) of jumbo rickrack in complimentary color to background
- ✓ Sewing machine and matching thread
- ✓ Note: This is a mostly no-sew project, but some rudimentary knowledge of sewing will help.

Directions:

1. Cut a rectangle measuring 20" × 30" from both pieces of fleece. One piece will be the front and the second color will be the back.
2. Cut out numbers 1 through 10 in contrasting color.
3. Draw a 10-square grid (2 horizontal rows of 5) on the front rectangle, as follows: Long sides are 5" from the top and bottom edges, short sides are 2½" from the side edges. Draw a horizontal line through the center of the rectangle. Mark off vertical lines every 5" starting with the left side and moving across to the right.
4. Line up the front and back rectangles, wrong sides together, and pin together along grid lines. Pins should be perpendicular to grid lines (so sewing machine can stitch over them).
5. Pin rickrack trim along grid lines and sew down using a wide zig-zag stitch.
6. Place the number "1" in the first grid box on the top row. Stitch around edges using open zig-zag stitch or straight stitch ⅛" from edge. Repeat with remaining numbers.
7. Make a channel to slip in a curtain rod for hanging. Stitch along upper edge of wall hanging, 3" down from top edge. This will create a 2" channel across the top of the rickrack to slide in a curtain rod for hanging it on the wall.
8. Sew on buttons in random placement for each number.
9. Create fringe. When all buttons are in place, lay wall hanging out flat. Using sharp scissors, cut top and bottom edges of fleece, through both layers, in 1" strips. Top fringe will be 3" long and bottom fridge will be 5" long. Tie each piece of front fringe to corresponding piece of back fringe to form a knot. Fringe should have a playful look.
10. Slip curtain rod through channel, attach finials, screw brackets into wall, and hang.

Chapter 13: Roses Kissed by Chocolate

This will make 2 dozen roses.

Materials Needed:

- ✓ 1 bag chocolate "kiss" candy
- ✓ 1 roll red foil or cellophane, cut into twenty-four 4" squares
- ✓ 2 packages medium-gauge (20–24 gauge) florist wire
- ✓ 1 roll florist tape
- ✓ 1 roll double-stick tape
- ✓ 3 dozen artificial leaves (optional—about 2 or 3 per rose)

- ✓ 12 yards ribbon (½ yard of ribbon per rose)
- ✓ Scissors
- ✓ Wire cutters
- ✓ Ruler and pen

Directions:

1. For each candy rose bud, begin by taping two kisses together, bottom to bottom.
2. Stick the florist wire into one end of the double chocolate (both ends are pointed).
3. Next, center 4" square of foil or cellophane around double chocolate, and cover the two kisses. Twist foil or cellophane tightly around chocolate kiss at the base.
4. Beginning at base of bud, wrap the florist tape tightly around edges of foil or cellophane and the florist wire. Continue down the length of wire with tape, adding one or two leaves about 3" down from the bud, until all the wire is covered. Break off at end.
5. Tie with ribbon and a tag with a note. "Bravo," "A Standing Ovation," or "A Kiss from Baby" could be inscribed on the tag.

Chapter 15: Chef Hats and Aprons

The chef's hat and matching apron are made using store-bought hats and aprons decorated with heat-transferred designs that you create and print on specialty paper from your computer. This technique is easy, requires only basic computer knowledge, and it's fun! See *www.everydayeventplanner.com* for ideas and designs.

Materials Needed:

- ✓ 1 chef's hat and 1 apron for each guest. Any color of apron will work. Typically, the chef hat only comes in white.
- ✓ 1 to 2 packages of iron-on T-shirt transfer paper for dark clothes. This is the best method for transferring images.
- ✓ 1 iron with high-heat setting
- ✓ Computer and printer access
- ✓ Hard surface to use for ironing clothing. A regular metal ironing board is not recommended by manufacturer.

Directions

1. Scan the design you wish to use into your computer. Make any adjustments you want to customize the look of your transfer design. When you are satisfied with the end product, print out onto specialty transfer paper. You should be able to get several images onto one transfer sheet.
2. Cut out around image and get ready to place.
3. Place the image where you want it on the apron or hat. Cover picture with the contact sheet that comes with the transfer paper.
4. Iron on designs as instructed by transfer-paper manufacturer.
5. You may embellish the aprons with fabric paints or just leave them as they are.

Appendix C

Templates for Customized Printing Projects

All templates are available online at *www.every dayeventplanner.com*.

Template for Theme Ideas Worksheet

When planning a shower with friends, some ideas sound like they would be fun, but then prove to be difficult to translate into décor, favors, and food. This worksheet can assist in determining which idea has the greatest chance for success.

Paint-Can Art

Gallon-can label size: $7\frac{1}{4}$" × 11"
Quart-can label: $4\frac{3}{4}$" × $7\frac{1}{2}$"

Directions:

1. Place information in center of label.
2. Print out or copy the number of labels needed.
3. Wrap label around can and secure label in place with double-sided tape.

Download this image from *www.everydayevent planner.com*.

Personalized Candy-Bar Label for Standard-Size Hershey's Candy Bars

Candy bar size $2\frac{1}{8}$" × $5\frac{1}{2}$"
Label size is $5\frac{1}{8}$" × $\frac{3}{8}$"

Directions:

1. Place information in center third of wrapper.
2. Print out or copy the number of labels needed.
3. Remove original label, leaving foil wrapper in place. Wrap with new label. (You can also leave original wrapper in place.)
4. Secure label in place with double-sided tape.

Download this image from *www.everydayevent planner.com*.

Binky Movie-Rating Sheet

Print out enough for each guest to get one sheet. As guests watch the chosen movie scenes, have them rate it by putting check marks for the numbers of binkies they feel it deserves. This is not an exact science—make up your own rules about what's good and bad!

Download this image from *www.everydayevent planner.com.*

Personalized CD-Case Label

Label Size is 4¾" x 4¾"

Directions:

1. Design CD-case label with shower information
2. Print out or copy the number of labels needed.
3. Cut out label and place in cover of standard-size CD case.

Download this image from *www.everydayevent planner.com.*

Personalized Favor-Bag Label

Label size is 4¾" × 4¾"

Directions:

1. Design favor bag label with shower information. Remember to arrange message on back upside down.
2. Print out or copy the number of labels needed.
3. Cut out, fold in half, and staple in bottom corners to cellophane bag full of goodies.

Download this image from *www.everydayevent planner.com.*

Index

Activities, 6, 73–82. *See also* Theme showers

Adoptions, 4

Allen, Amy, 102

Appetizers, 15

Art activities, 79–80

Artistic-theme shower, 206–8

At-home showers, 11–12, 15, 18–19, 53, 108, 112, 114, 135, 138

At-work showers, 10, 12, 213–17

Baby Back Barbeque Short Ribs, 263

"Baby Bingo," 75

Baby clothes, 29, 33, 68, 87–88, 102, 196

"Baby Diapering Game," 74

Baby feeding activity, 78

Baby foods, 78–79

Baby furniture, 88–89

Baby gifts. *See* Gifts; Theme gifts

"Baby Grand Piano" shower, 154–56

Baby massage, 77–78

"Baby Picasso," 76

Baby pictures games, 76

"Baby Pins in a Bottle," 76

"Baby Quilt" activity, 79–80

"Baby" Red Potatoes, 259

Baby showers. *See also* Theme showers
beginning and ending, 4–7

history of, xiii

hostess of, 2–4, 87

length of, 3, 12

number of, 3

planning, xiii–xiv, 1–23, 27

scheduling, 2, 10–12

Baby talk, 85

Baby themes, 29–30. *See also* Theme showers

Baby toys, 29, 33, 64, 89

"Baby Trivia," 74

Bacharach, Burt, 106

Bath themes, 33

Beach showers, 21–22

Beauty product favors, 71–72

Beefsteak Tomatoes and Onions, 266

"Belly Bump" shower
menu for, 129
recipes for, 243–47
theme for, 128–31

Bennett, Tony, 106

Beverages, 5, 17–18, 50

"Birthday Card" activity, 82

Biscotti, 268–69

Black Bottom Cupcakes, 273

Blue Corn Chips and Chunky Guacamole, 257

"Book Collection" shower, 138–40

Breakfast, 18, 49

Breakfast martini, 50

Bright Chili Beans, 224

Broadway baby showers

    menu for, 148

    recipes for, 250–51

    theme for, 145–56

Brownie Bar with Candy Bar Toppings, 225

Brunch, 18, 50

Budget, 12–13, 17, 63

Budget-planning worksheet, 13

Buffet, 47–48, 52

Build-a-Burger Barbeque, 95–96

Butterscotch Sauce, 255

"Button" cupcakes, 115

Caesar Salad, 248

Cake Mix Cookies, 262

Cake recipes, 236, 249

Cakes, 15, 50, 52, 68, 84, 110, 136

Calendar themes, 33–34

Carrot and Parsnip with Ginger, 227

Caterers, 14, 16, 18, 22, 55–57

"Celebrity Baby Pictures," 76

Celebrity-style showers

    menu for, 103

recipes for, 222–34

    theme for, 93–106

Centerpieces, 66–68. *See also* Theme
  showers

Chai Tea Mix, 243

Cheesecake, 267

Chicken Curry, 244

Chicken with Rice, 271

Chilled Tomato Soup with Guacamole,
  227–28

Chocolate Butter Rum Truffles, 233–34

Chocolate Fondue, 251

Chocolate Shortbread, 230

Chocolate Yummies, 270

Chuck Wagon Cornbread, 266

Chuck Wagon Kidney Beans, 265

Cilantro Chicken Dumplings, 240

Classic Asparagus with Lemon and Olive Oil,
  232

Classic Reuben Sandwich, 261

Classic Swiss Cheese Fondue, 250

Cocktail parties, 5, 18, 34, 47, 51, 77, 105

Coffee Almond Float in Espresso Cups, 229

Coffee breaks, 18, 210, 213–17

"Coffee Break" shower

    menu for, 215–16

    recipes for, 268–70

    theme for, 213–17

Coffee Cake, 269–70

Cohosts, 8, 11, 14, 27–28

Color schemes, 26, 29, 39–40, 64–66. *See also* Theme showers

Cookie-Cutter French Toast, 238–39

Costs, 12–13, 17

Costs worksheet, 13

Couples' cocktail parties, 18, 34, 51, 77, 105

Couples' showers, 69, 103–6, 157–68. *See also* Jack and Jill showers

Couric, Katie, 102

Craft activities, 79–80

Crustless Quiche Lorraine, 239

Crystal, Billy, 102

Cupcakes, 15, 41, 52, 68, 115, 273

Curtis, Jamie Lee, 102

"Cute as a Button" shower
  menu for, 114
  recipes for, 237
  theme for, 114–16

Daddy gear, 86

Dads' showers
  menu for, 187, 190, 194
  recipes for, 261–67
  theme for, 183–96

Date, choosing, 10–12

Décor. *See also* Theme showers
  basics of, 58–72
  budget for, 63
  celebrity-style décor, 94–95
  and centerpieces, 66–68
  and color, 64–66
  elements of, 60–64
  ideas for, 6, 15–16, 62–63, 66–69
  and napkin rings, 68–69
  and shower needs, 63–64

Demographics, 10, 30

"Desktop" showers, 213–17

Desserts, 15, 18, 41, 52, 84, 110, 115, 136, 148, 173

Destination showers, 21–22

Diaper cake, 68

Diaper games, 74

Diapers, 88

"Diapers Wild!" shower
  menu for, 159
  recipes for, 252–53
  theme for, 158–62

"Digital Daddy" showers, 186–90

Dinners, 18, 51–52

Drama Buff showers, 145–56

Dry-Spiced Carrots and Peas, 246–47

Egba Party Block, 94

Eggplant Caviar, 230

Entertainment tips, 6, 15–16

E-showers

   menu for, 215, 217

   recipes for, 268–73

   theme for, 209–20

Espresso Truffles, 234

Estelle's Cream-Cheese Pound Cake, 249

Etiquette, 2–4, 210, 214

Evite.com, 37

Expenses, 12–13, 17

"Extreme Nursery Makeover" shower

   menu for, 190

   recipes for, 261–62

   theme for, 190–93

Fashionable themes, 31–32

Fashion clothes, 86–87, 99, 198–203

Favors, 69–72. *See also* Theme showers

Feeding activity, 78

Foods. *See also* Menus; Recipes

   to avoid, 49

   baby foods, 78–79

   costs of, 17

   as favors, 70–71

   ideas for, 6, 15, 17–18

presentation of, 53–54

rules about, 48–49, 52–53

tips on, 15, 45–48

Food service, 46–48

Food stations, 19, 48, 55

"Footsie, Tootsie" shower

   menu for, 109–10

   recipes for, 235–36

   theme for, 109–14

Formality, degree of, 10

Fourth of July–Ade, 222

Fresh Scones, 268

Fried Bowties, 242

Furniture for nursery, 88–89

Game prizes, 75, 77, 116, 124, 162, 165

Games, 6, 73–82. *See also* Theme showers

Garden Pea Couscous Salad with Roasted

   Chicken Breast, 228

Garlic Bread, 248

German Potato Salad, 224–25

Get Your Snack Mixer On, 223

Gift certificates, 84, 85, 210, 211, 216. *See also*

   Gifts

Gift registry, 91–92. *See also* Gifts

Gifts. *See also* Theme gifts

   ideas for, xiv, 83–92

opening, 3, 6, 84–85

personalized gifts, 90–91, 138, 213

registry for, 91–92

and thank-you notes, 3–4, 6–7, 84–85

tracking, 84–85

traditional gifts, 87–89

trendy gifts, 85–87

wrappings for, 84

Ginger-Garlic Paste, 245

"Girlfriends Go Wild" showers

menu for, 109–10, 114, 117

recipes for, 235–39

theme for, 106–18

Girls' night out, 34

Grandma's Beef Stew, 247–48

Grandparents' showers

menu for, 136

recipes for, 247–49

theme for, 133–44

Gratitude, 6–7. See also Thank-you notes

Gratuities, 16

Greek Salad, 260

"Green" baby gifts, 85

Grilled Pears with Claret Sauce, 233

Group planning tips, 8

Guessing games, 75–76

Guest list, 36. See also Invitations

Guests, 5–7, 10, 30

Gutter Ball Subs, 254

Helen's Dulce de Leche Fondue, 251

"Hello Dolly!" shower, 151–52

Herb-Crusted Salmon, 231

Hobby themes, 32

Hollywood trends, 93–94, 103, 106. See also
   Celebrity-style showers

Home showers, 11–12, 15, 18–19, 53, 108, 112,
   114, 135, 138

Hostess, 2–4, 87. See also Cohosts

Hot and Sweet Italian Sausage, 258

Hotels, xiii, 11, 15–20. See also Venues

Hot Fudge Sauce, 255

Hummus, 258

Icebreakers, 6

Ice-Cream Sandwiches, 253

Introductions, 6

Invitations. See also Theme invitations

budget for, 12

designs for, 41–43, 94

fonts for, 40–41

and guest list, 36

hand-crafting, 43
ideas for, 35–44
information for, 37–38
options for, 35–44
postage for, 44
and R.S.V.P.s, 37–39
special effects for, 43–44
types of, xiv, 5, 26, 36–37
Italian Sub Sandwiches, 252
Itineraries, 5

Jack and Jill showers
menu for, 159, 163, 166
recipes for, 252–56
theme for, 157–68
John, Elton, 106
Jones, Norah, 106

Keepsakes, 90–91, 138, 213
Kingpin Coleslaw, 254

"Lap-top" showers
menu for, 217
recipes for, 270–73
theme for, 217–20

Last trimester, 10–11, 86, 198, 201–2
Layette, 29, 33, 68, 87–88, 102, 196
Limeade, 256
Lithgow, John, 102
Location for showers, xiii, 11, 15–23, 26,
108, 131–32, 135, 199. *See also* Hotels;
Restaurants
"Lucky Strike!" shower
menu for, 163
recipes for, 254–55
theme for, 162–65
Lunch, 18, 50

Macaroni Salad, 262
Madonna, 102
Main course, 15, 50, 172
Malabari Coconut Rice, 246
Martin, Michelle, 40
"Mary, Mary, Quite Contrary," 75
Maternity clothes, 86, 99, 200–203
Memory-making activities, 81–82. *See also*
Keepsakes
Men, and showers, 30, 50, 69, 134, 157–68,
183–96. *See also* Couples' cocktail parties
Menus. *See also* Foods; Recipes
for appetizers, 15
basics of, 45–57

for breakfast, 49

Broadway theme, 147–48

for brunch, 50

for buffets, 47–48, 52

and caterers, 55–57

celebrity-style themes, 95–96, 100, 103

for cocktail parties, 51

coffee break theme, 215–16

couples theme, 159

dads theme, 187, 190, 194

for desserts, 15, 52

for dinner, 51–52

girlfriends theme, 109–10, 114, 117

grandparents theme, 136

for lunch, 50

for main course, 15

neighborly theme, 173

planning ahead for, 54–55

road rally theme, 166

rules for, 48–49, 52–53

tailgate theme, 194

tea theme, 50–51, 121–23, 129, 131–32

urban baby theme, 200

workplace theme, 215–17

Mexican Hot Chocolate, 238

Minimalist showers, 34

Minted Pea Soup, 226

Miso Soup Shots, 240

"Mocktails," 50

Money-savers, 14

Monthly themes, 33–34

"Mother's Circumference," 76

Movie themes, 30–32

Multiple babies, 4

Multiple showers, 3

Music, 6

Myths, xii

Nametags, 5

Napkin rings, 68–69

Neighborly showers

menu for, 173

recipes for, 256–61

theme for, 169–82

"Night-Night" shower

menu for, 117

recipes for, 238–39

theme for, 116–18

Nursery furnishings, 88–89

Online invitation sites, 37

Oven-Fried Chicken Nuggets, 272

"Painted Canvas Baby Quilt," 79–80

Painting activities, 79–80

"Parenting Advice Book," 82

Parmesan Crisps, 229

Party favors, 69–72

Party framework, 4–7

Party themes. *See* Theme showers

Pedicure shower, 109–14

Personalized gifts, 90–91, 138, 213

Phair, Liz, 106

Pink Ladies'-Ade, 237

"Pin the Diaper on the Baby," 74

Planning tips, xiii–xiv, 1–23, 27. *See also*
  Theme showers

Planning tools, 9–23

Pomegranate Chaat, 247

Pop culture themes, 30–31

Porter, Cole, 106

Post, Emily, 4

Potato Salad with Egg, 253

Pound Cake, 249

Presents. *See* Gifts

"Price Is Right Game," 75–76

"Princess Wears Prada" shower
  menu for, 100
  recipes for, 225–30
  theme for, 99–102

Printing project templates, 289–90

Prizes, 75, 77, 116, 124, 162, 165

Professional help, 14

Project directions, 285–90

Quickie Pasta Bake, 271–72

Raspberry Coulis, 249

Real Macaroni and Cheese, 272–73

Recipes, 221–73

"Red Carpet" showers
  menu for, 103
  recipes for, 230–34
  theme for, 103–6

"Red Wagon" showers
  menu for, 173
  recipes for, 256–61
  theme for, 170–82

Rental contract, 20, 57

Rental supplies, 19

Resources, 275–83

Restaurants, xiii, 11–12, 15–20, 50, 57, 131–32,
  135. *See also* Venues

"Road Rally" shower
  menu for, 166

recipes for, 256

theme for, 165–68

Rose Lemonade with Rose Petals, 226

Saffron Lemonade, 243

Salad Bar recipes, 235–36

Salon showers, 21–22

Salsa recipe, 28

"Save a Bundle" shower, 141–44

"Scrapbook-Making" shower, 81

Self-service meals, 47–48

Serving styles, 46–48

Shower games, 6, 73–82. *See also* Theme showers

Shower ideas. *See* Baby showers; Theme showers

Shower locations, xiii, 11, 15–23, 26, 108, 131–32, 135, 199. *See also* Hotels; Restaurants

Shower recipes, 221–73

Shrimp and Green Onion Dumplings, 241

Shrimp Crab Dip, 257

Sign language, 85

Sirloin, Round, and Chuck Burger, 223–24

Smoked Turkey Salad, 237

Snacks, 6, 70–71. *See also* Foods

Spa showers, 21–22, 27, 75, 77, 108–9, 120

Specialty showers, 21–22. *See also* Theme showers

Spicy Barbeque Sauce, 264

Spicy-Tart Apple Sauce, 259

Spring Rolls, 241–42

Stonepine Iced Tea, 247

Strawberry Lemonade, 235

Strawberry Shortcake, 260–61

Stress-savers, 14

Stuffed Filet Mignon, 231–32

Surprise showers, 2

Surrogate births, 4

"Tailgate" showers

menu for, 194

recipes for, 263–67

theme for, 193–96

Tasseography, 125–27

"Tea" showers

menu for, 121–23, 128

recipes for, 240–46

theme for, 50–51, 119–32

"Teddy Bear Workshop," 80

Templates, 289–90

Texas Sheet Cake, 236

Thank-you notes, 3–4, 6–7, 84–85

Theme gifts. *See also* Gifts
 bowling theme, 164
 Broadway theme, 150, 153, 155
 celebrity-style themes, 98, 102, 106
 couples theme, 162
 dads theme, 189–90, 193, 196
 e-shower theme, 213
 fashion theme, 203, 205, 208
 first visit theme, 219–20
 girlfriends theme, 113, 116, 118
 grandparents theme, 140, 143–44
 ideas for, 33–34, 89–90
 neighborly theme, 174, 178–79
 road rally theme, 168
 tea theme, 127, 130, 132
 urban baby theme, 203–5, 208
 workplace theme, 216
Theme invitations. *See also* Invitations
 bowling theme, 163
 Broadway theme, 148
 celebrity-style themes, 97, 101, 105, 109
 couples theme, 159
 dads theme, 185–86
 e-shower theme, 214
 girlfriends theme, 109
 grandparents theme, 136–37, 139, 141–42
 neighborly theme, 172, 177–78

 road rally theme, 166
 tea theme, 123, 128
 urban baby theme, 199
 workplace theme, 214
Theme showers. *See also* Menus
 Broadway theme, 145–56
 celebrity-style themes, 93–106
 choosing, 21–23, 25–34
 couples theme, 157–68
 dads theme, 183–96
 e-shower theme, 209–20
 girlfriends theme, 107–18
 grandparents theme, 133–44
 ideas for, 21–23, 25–34
 neighborly theme, 169–82
 tea theme, 119–32
 urban baby theme, 197–208
Three-dimensional invitations, 94
Time for shower, 10–12
Timesavers, 17
Tortilla Lasagna, 270
Tour-theme shower, 203–6
Toys, 29, 33, 64, 69, 89
Traffic flow, 19, 48, 57, 61
Trail Mix, 256
"Tranquili-Tea" shower
 menu for, 121–22

recipes for, 240–42

theme for, 121–23

Travel themes, 33

TV themes, 30–31

Yukon Gold Potatoes with Oregano, 232

"Under Construction" shower

menu for, 95–96

recipes for, 222–25

theme for, 95–99

Urban baby showers, 197–208

"Zen Tea" showers

menu for, 121–23, 128

recipes for, 240–46

theme for, 119–32

Vanderbilt, Amy, 3–4

Venue checklist, 22–23

Venues, xiii, 11, 15–23, 26, 108, 131–32, 135, 199. *See also* Hotels; Restaurants

Virtual showers

menu for, 215, 217

recipes for, 268–73

theme for, 209–20

Warm Spice Mix, 244

Weekend showers, 11–12

"Welcome Station," 5–6

"Who's Who Baby Pictures Game," 76

THE EVERYTHING SERIES!

BUSINESS & PERSONAL FINANCE

Everything® Accounting Book
Everything® Budgeting Book
Everything® Business Planning Book
Everything® Coaching and Mentoring Book
Everything® Fundraising Book
Everything® Get Out of Debt Book
Everything® Grant Writing Book
Everything® Guide to Personal Finance for Single Mothers
Everything® Home-Based Business Book, 2nd Ed.
Everything® Homebuying Book, 2nd Ed.
Everything® Homeselling Book, 2nd Ed.
Everything® Improve Your Credit Book
Everything® Investing Book, 2nd Ed.
Everything® Landlording Book
Everything® Leadership Book
Everything® Managing People Book, 2nd Ed.
Everything® Negotiating Book
Everything® Online Auctions Book
Everything® Online Business Book
Everything® Personal Finance Book
Everything® Personal Finance in Your 20s and 30s Book
Everything® Project Management Book
Everything® Real Estate Investing Book
Everything® Retirement Planning Book
Everything® Robert's Rules Book, $7.95
Everything® Selling Book
Everything® Start Your Own Business Book, 2nd Ed.
Everything® Wills & Estate Planning Book

COOKING

Everything® Barbecue Cookbook
Everything® Bartender's Book, $9.95
Everything® Cheese Book
Everything® Chinese Cookbook
Everything® Classic Recipes Book
Everything® Cocktail Parties and Drinks Book
Everything® College Cookbook
Everything® Cooking for Baby and Toddler Book
Everything® Cooking for Two Cookbook
Everything® Diabetes Cookbook
Everything® Easy Gourmet Cookbook
Everything® Fondue Cookbook
Everything® Fondue Party Book
Everything® Gluten-Free Cookbook
Everything® Glycemic Index Cookbook
Everything® Grilling Cookbook

Everything® Healthy Meals in Minutes Cookbook
Everything® Holiday Cookbook
Everything® Indian Cookbook
Everything® Italian Cookbook
Everything® Low-Carb Cookbook
Everything® Low-Fat High-Flavor Cookbook
Everything® Low-Salt Cookbook
Everything® Meals for a Month Cookbook
Everything® Mediterranean Cookbook
Everything® Mexican Cookbook
Everything® No Trans Fat Cookbook
Everything® One-Pot Cookbook
Everything® Pizza Cookbook
Everything® Quick and Easy 30-Minute, 5-Ingredient Cookbook
Everything® Quick Meals Cookbook
Everything® Slow Cooker Cookbook
Everything® Slow Cooking for a Crowd Cookbook
Everything® Soup Cookbook
Everything® Stir-Fry Cookbook
Everything® Tex-Mex Cookbook
Everything® Thai Cookbook
Everything® Vegetarian Cookbook
Everything® Wild Game Cookbook
Everything® Wine Book, 2nd Ed.

GAMES

Everything® 15-Minute Sudoku Book, $9.95
Everything® 30-Minute Sudoku Book, $9.95
Everything® Blackjack Strategy Book
Everything® Brain Strain Book, $9.95
Everything® Bridge Book
Everything® Card Games Book
Everything® Card Tricks Book, $9.95
Everything® Casino Gambling Book, 2nd Ed.
Everything® Chess Basics Book
Everything® Craps Strategy Book
Everything® Crossword and Puzzle Book
Everything® Crossword Challenge Book
Everything® Crosswords for the Beach Book, $9.95
Everything® Cryptograms Book, $9.95
Everything® Easy Crosswords Book
Everything® Easy Kakuro Book, $9.95
Everything® Easy Large Print Crosswords Book
Everything® Games Book, 2nd Ed.
Everything® Giant Sudoku Book, $9.95
Everything® Kakuro Challenge Book, $9.95
Everything® Large-Print Crossword Challenge Book

Everything® Large-Print Crosswords Book
Everything® Lateral Thinking Puzzles Book, $9.95
Everything® Mazes Book
Everything® Movie Crosswords Book, $9.95
Everything® Online Poker Book, $12.95
Everything® Pencil Puzzles Book, $9.95
Everything® Poker Strategy Book
Everything® Pool & Billiards Book
Everything® Sports Crosswords Book, $9.95
Everything® Test Your IQ Book, $9.95
Everything® Texas Hold 'Em Book, $9.95
Everything® Travel Crosswords Book, $9.95
Everything® Word Games Challenge Book
Everything® Word Scramble Book
Everything® Word Search Book

HEALTH

Everything® Alzheimer's Book
Everything® Diabetes Book
Everything® Health Guide to Adult Bipolar Disorder
Everything® Health Guide to Controlling Anxiety
Everything® Health Guide to Fibromyalgia
Everything® Health Guide to Postpartum Care
Everything® Health Guide to Thyroid Disease
Everything® Hypnosis Book
Everything® Low Cholesterol Book
Everything® Massage Book
Everything® Menopause Book
Everything® Nutrition Book
Everything® Reflexology Book
Everything® Stress Management Book

HISTORY

Everything® American Government Book
Everything® American History Book, 2nd Ed.
Everything® Civil War Book
Everything® Freemasons Book
Everything® Irish History & Heritage Book
Everything® Middle East Book

HOBBIES

Everything® Candlemaking Book
Everything® Cartooning Book
Everything® Coin Collecting Book
Everything® Drawing Book
Everything® Family Tree Book, 2nd Ed.
Everything® Knitting Book
Everything® Knots Book
Everything® Photography Book

Everything® Quilting Book
Everything® Scrapbooking Book
Everything® Sewing Book
Everything® Soapmaking Book, 2nd Ed.
Everything® Woodworking Book

HOME IMPROVEMENT

Everything® Feng Shui Book
Everything® Feng Shui Decluttering Book, $9.95
Everything® Fix-It Book
Everything® Home Decorating Book
Everything® Home Storage Solutions Book
Everything® Homebuilding Book
Everything® Organize Your Home Book

KIDS' BOOKS

All titles are $7.95
Everything® Kids' Animal Puzzle & Activity Book
Everything® Kids' Baseball Book, 4th Ed.
Everything® Kids' Bible Trivia Book
Everything® Kids' Bugs Book
Everything® Kids' Cars and Trucks Puzzle & Activity Book
Everything® Kids' Christmas Puzzle & Activity Book
Everything® Kids' Cookbook
Everything® Kids' Crazy Puzzles Book
Everything® Kids' Dinosaurs Book
Everything® Kids' First Spanish Puzzle and Activity Book
Everything® Kids' Gross Cookbook
Everything® Kids' Gross Hidden Pictures Book
Everything® Kids' Gross Jokes Book
Everything® Kids' Gross Mazes Book
Everything® Kids' Gross Puzzle and Activity Book
Everything® Kids' Halloween Puzzle & Activity Book
Everything® Kids' Hidden Pictures Book
Everything® Kids' Horses Book
Everything® Kids' Joke Book
Everything® Kids' Knock Knock Book
Everything® Kids' Learning Spanish Book
Everything® Kids' Math Puzzles Book
Everything® Kids' Mazes Book
Everything® Kids' Money Book
Everything® Kids' Nature Book
Everything® Kids' Pirates Puzzle and Activity Book
Everything® Kids' Presidents Book
Everything® Kids' Princess Puzzle and Activity Book
Everything® Kids' Puzzle Book
Everything® Kids' Riddles & Brain Teasers Book
Everything® Kids' Science Experiments Book
Everything® Kids' Sharks Book
Everything® Kids' Soccer Book
Everything® Kids' States Book
Everything® Kids' Travel Activity Book

KIDS' STORY BOOKS

Everything® Fairy Tales Book

LANGUAGE

Everything® Conversational Japanese Book with CD, $19.95
Everything® French Grammar Book
Everything® French Phrase Book, $9.95
Everything® French Verb Book, $9.95
Everything® German Practice Book with CD, $19.95
Everything® Inglés Book
Everything® Intermediate Spanish Book with CD, $19.95
Everything® Learning Brazilian Portuguese Book with CD, $19.95
Everything® Learning French Book
Everything® Learning German Book
Everything® Learning Italian Book
Everything® Learning Latin Book
Everything® Learning Spanish Book with CD, 2nd Edition, $19.95
Everything® Russian Practice Book with CD, $19.95
Everything® Sign Language Book
Everything® Spanish Grammar Book
Everything® Spanish Phrase Book, $9.95
Everything® Spanish Practice Book with CD, $19.95
Everything® Spanish Verb Book, $9.95
Everything® Speaking Mandarin Chinese Book with CD, $19.95

MUSIC

Everything® Drums Book with CD, $19.95
Everything® Guitar Book with CD, 2nd Edition, $19.95
Everything® Guitar Chords Book with CD, $19.95
Everything® Home Recording Book
Everything® Music Theory Book with CD, $19.95
Everything® Reading Music Book with CD, $19.95
Everything® Rock & Blues Guitar Book with CD, $19.95
Everything® Rock and Blues Piano Book with CD, $19.95
Everything® Songwriting Book

NEW AGE

Everything® Astrology Book, 2nd Ed.
Everything® Birthday Personology Book
Everything® Dreams Book, 2nd Ed.
Everything® Love Signs Book, $9.95
Everything® Numerology Book
Everything® Paganism Book
Everything® Palmistry Book
Everything® Psychic Book
Everything® Reiki Book

Everything® Sex Signs Book, $9.95
Everything® Tarot Book, 2nd Ed.
Everything® Toltec Wisdom Book
Everything® Wicca and Witchcraft Book

PARENTING

Everything® Baby Names Book, 2nd Ed.
Everything® Baby Shower Book
Everything® Baby's First Year Book
Everything® Birthing Book
Everything® Breastfeeding Book
Everything® Father-to-Be Book
Everything® Father's First Year Book
Everything® Get Ready for Baby Book
Everything® Get Your Baby to Sleep Book, $9.95
Everything® Getting Pregnant Book
Everything® Guide to Raising a One-Year-Old
Everything® Guide to Raising a Two-Year-Old
Everything® Homeschooling Book
Everything® Mother's First Year Book
Everything® Parent's Guide to Childhood Illnesses
Everything® Parent's Guide to Children and Divorce
Everything® Parent's Guide to Children with ADD/ADHD
Everything® Parent's Guide to Children with Asperger's Syndrome
Everything® Parent's Guide to Children with Autism
Everything® Parent's Guide to Children with Bipolar Disorder
Everything® Parent's Guide to Children with Depression
Everything® Parent's Guide to Children with Dyslexia
Everything® Parent's Guide to Children with Juvenile Diabetes
Everything® Parent's Guide to Positive Discipline
Everything® Parent's Guide to Raising a Successful Child
Everything® Parent's Guide to Raising Boys
Everything® Parent's Guide to Raising Girls
Everything® Parent's Guide to Raising Siblings
Everything® Parent's Guide to Sensory Integration Disorder
Everything® Parent's Guide to Tantrums
Everything® Parent's Guide to the Strong-Willed Child
Everything® Parenting a Teenager Book
Everything® Potty Training Book, $9.95
Everything® Pregnancy Book, 3rd Ed.
Everything® Pregnancy Fitness Book
Everything® Pregnancy Nutrition Book
Everything® Pregnancy Organizer, 2nd Ed., $16.95
Everything® Toddler Activities Book
Everything® Toddler Book

Everything® Tween Book
Everything® Twins, Triplets, and More Book

PETS

Everything® Aquarium Book
Everything® Boxer Book
Everything® Cat Book, 2nd Ed.
Everything® Chihuahua Book
Everything® Dachshund Book
Everything® Dog Book
Everything® Dog Health Book
Everything® Dog Obedience Book
Everything® Dog Owner's Organizer, $16.95
Everything® Dog Training and Tricks Book
Everything® German Shepherd Book
Everything® Golden Retriever Book
Everything® Horse Book
Everything® Horse Care Book
Everything® Horseback Riding Book
Everything® Labrador Retriever Book
Everything® Poodle Book
Everything® Pug Book
Everything® Puppy Book
Everything® Rottweiler Book
Everything® Small Dogs Book
Everything® Tropical Fish Book
Everything® Yorkshire Terrier Book

REFERENCE

Everything® American Presidents Book
Everything® Blogging Book
Everything® Build Your Vocabulary Book
Everything® Car Care Book
Everything® Classical Mythology Book
Everything® Da Vinci Book
Everything® Divorce Book
Everything® Einstein Book
Everything® Enneagram Book
Everything® Etiquette Book, 2nd Ed.
Everything® Inventions and Patents Book
Everything® Mafia Book
Everything® Philosophy Book
Everything® Pirates Book
Everything® Psychology Book

RELIGION

Everything® Angels Book
Everything® Bible Book
Everything® Buddhism Book
Everything® Catholicism Book
Everything® Christianity Book
Everything® Gnostic Gospels Book
Everything® History of the Bible Book
Everything® Jesus Book

Everything® Jewish History & Heritage Book
Everything® Judaism Book
Everything® Kabbalah Book
Everything® Koran Book
Everything® Mary Book
Everything® Mary Magdalene Book
Everything® Prayer Book
Everything® Saints Book, 2nd Ed.
Everything® Torah Book
Everything® Understanding Islam Book
Everything® World's Religions Book
Everything® Zen Book

SCHOOL & CAREERS

Everything® Alternative Careers Book
Everything® Career Tests Book
Everything® College Major Test Book
Everything® College Survival Book, 2nd Ed.
Everything® Cover Letter Book, 2nd Ed.
Everything® Filmmaking Book
Everything® Get-a-Job Book, 2nd Ed.
Everything® Guide to Being a Paralegal
Everything® Guide to Being a Personal Trainer
Everything® Guide to Being a Real Estate Agent
Everything® Guide to Being a Sales Rep
Everything® Guide to Careers in Health Care
Everything® Guide to Careers in Law Enforcement
Everything® Guide to Government Jobs
Everything® Guide to Starting and Running a Restaurant
Everything® Job Interview Book
Everything® New Nurse Book
Everything® New Teacher Book
Everything® Paying for College Book
Everything® Practice Interview Book
Everything® Resume Book, 2nd Ed.
Everything® Study Book

SELF-HELP

Everything® Dating Book, 2nd Ed.
Everything® Great Sex Book
Everything® Self-Esteem Book
Everything® Tantric Sex Book

SPORTS & FITNESS

Everything® Easy Fitness Book
Everything® Running Book
Everything® Weight Training Book

TRAVEL

Everything® Family Guide to Cruise Vacations
Everything® Family Guide to Hawaii
Everything® Family Guide to Las Vegas, 2nd Ed.
Everything® Family Guide to Mexico
Everything® Family Guide to New York City, 2nd Ed.
Everything® Family Guide to RV Travel & Campgrounds
Everything® Family Guide to the Caribbean
Everything® Family Guide to the Walt Disney World Resort®, Universal Studios®, and Greater Orlando, 4th Ed.
Everything® Family Guide to Timeshares
Everything® Family Guide to Washington D.C., 2nd Ed.

WEDDINGS

Everything® Bachelorette Party Book, $9.95
Everything® Bridesmaid Book, $9.95
Everything® Destination Wedding Book
Everything® Elopement Book, $9.95
Everything® Father of the Bride Book, $9.95
Everything® Groom Book, $9.95
Everything® Mother of the Bride Book, $9.95
Everything® Outdoor Wedding Book
Everything® Wedding Book, 3rd Ed.
Everything® Wedding Checklist, $9.95
Everything® Wedding Etiquette Book, $9.95
Everything® Wedding Organizer, 2nd Ed., $16.95
Everything® Wedding Shower Book, $9.95
Everything® Wedding Vows Book, $9.95
Everything® Wedding Workout Book
Everything® Weddings on a Budget Book, $9.95

WRITING

Everything® Creative Writing Book
Everything® Get Published Book, 2nd Ed.
Everything® Grammar and Style Book
Everything® Guide to Magazine Writing
Everything® Guide to Writing a Book Proposal
Everything® Guide to Writing a Novel
Everything® Guide to Writing Children's Books
Everything® Guide to Writing Copy
Everything® Guide to Writing Research Papers
Everything® Screenwriting Book
Everything® Writing Poetry Book
Everything® Writing Well Book